When properly conducted, rou
ally challenging exercise for all involved. This book captures some of
that atmosphere—you'll enjoy it.

David E. Rogers
The Walsh McDermott University Professor of Medicine
Cornell University Medical College

One of the major challenges of medical (and graduate) school is to guide students through the transition from a dependence on textbooks to reading the literature. *Roundsmanship* should assist this transition.

William R. Hendee, Ph.D.
Vice President for Science and Technology
American Medical Association

This was a brilliant idea and the choice of editor is a good one. I hope gifted teachers will submit vignettes and pearls to the editor for inclusion in future volumes.

John Bergan, M.D., F.A.C.S., Hon. F.R.C.S. (Eng.)
Clinical Professor of Surgery
University of California, San Diego

I think it will be a very valuable book for house staff and others wishing to keep abreast of the entire spectrum of medicine. Even to medical subspecialists it offers the opportunity for them to see the highlights of other areas of medicine. The editor's comments on the specific article, as well as the "pearls," are helpful and are written in a style likely to make them remembered.

Robert C. Young, M.D.
President
Fox Chase Cancer Center

It seems to me to be a marvelous concept and to have been executed very well. The editors and topics are well chosen and the book is delightful to read.

Byron J. Bailey
Weiss Professor and Chairman
The University of Texas Medical Branch at Galveston

Editor-in-Chief

Bruce B. Dan, M.D.
Senior Editor, The Journal of the American Medical Association, Chicago

Editors

Ralph D. Feigin, M.D.
J.S. Abercrombie Professor and Chairman, Department of Pediatrics, Baylor College of Medicine, Houston, and Physician-in-Chief, Texas Children's Hospital

Edward J. Quilligan, M.D.
Professor of Obstetrics and Gynecology, University of California, Irvine

Seymour I. Schwartz, M.D.
Professor and Chair, Department of Surgery, University of Rochester School of Medicine and Dentistry

Jay H. Stein, M.D.
Professor and Chairman, Dan F. Parman Chair in Medicine, Department of Medicine, The University of Texas Health Sciences Center at San Antonio

John A. Talbott, M.D.
Professor and Chairman, Department of Psychiatry, University of Maryland School of Medicine; Director, Institute of Psychiatry and Human Behavior, University of Maryland Medical Systems, Baltimore

With an original introductory article by:

Robert G. Petersdorf, M.D.
President, Association of American Medical Colleges, Washington, D.C.

Roundsmanship '90: A YEAR BOOK® Guide to Clinical Medicine

Editor-in-Chief
Bruce B. Dan, M.D.

Editors
Ralph D. Feigin, M.D.
Edward J. Quilligan, M.D.
Seymour I. Schwartz, M.D.
Jay H. Stein, M.D.
John A. Talbott, M.D.

Year Book Medical Publishers, Inc.
Chicago • London • Boca Raton • Littleton, Mass.

Printed in U.S.A.

International Standard Book Number: 0-8151-2304-3

International Standard Serial Number: 1040–8487

Editor-in-Chief, Year Book Publishing: Nancy Gorham

Sponsoring Editors: Cara D. Suber and Sharon Tehan

Senior Medical Information Specialist: Terri Strorigl

Assistant Director, Manuscript Services: Frances M. Perveiler

Associate Managing Editor: Elizabeth Fitch

Production Coordinator: Max F. Perez

Proofroom Supervisor: Barbara M. Kelly

TABLE OF CONTENTS

Acknowledgment

Although only six names appear on the cover of *Roundsmanship,* all of the pages in between come from the diligent work of a number of people. Credit for the book and thanks as well are due the following individuals who make *Roundsmanship* what it is: David Cramer, M.D., for his major work in writing the abstracts, Terri Strorigl for coordinating the mammoth literature surveillance, and Max Perez for putting it all on paper. The Year Book editorial team of Nancy Gorham, Cara Suber, and Sharon Tehan deserves recognition, too, as the behind-the-scene editors, whose work is quite visible and who find, place, and even create the missing pieces to the "puzzle."

DEDICATION

Roundsmanship '90 is dedicated to the memory of Stephen R. Preblud, M.D. (1948–1989), Chief of the Surveillance, Investigations and Research Branch of the Division of Immunization at the Centers for Disease Control. Dr. Preblud was an acknowledged international authority on rubella, varicella, and mumps, and made landmark contributions to the understanding and prevention of childhood diseases. He was largely responsible for the control and elimination of rubella and congenital rubella syndrome both in the United States and abroad. His contributions to medicine over a short span were accomplishments to be proud of when achieved over a lifetime career. A teacher, researcher, and physician, Steve will be missed by his friends and by the millions of children around the world whose quality of life he helped improve, most of whom will have never heard his name.

Bruce B. Dan, M.D.

It is not to be imagined that he should know the remedy of diseases who knows not their original cause.

—Hippocrates

INTRODUCTION

'Round, 'round, get around, I get around . . . .
The Beach Boys, 1964

Like rounds themselves, *Roundsmanship* has come around again. *Roundsmanship '90* is the second edition of our series; our attempt to capture in one place, the most important articles published in the medical literature during the past year. We've again gathered together an impressive group of academic physicians who have chosen the articles and commented on why they believe they're so essential. While these short abstracts and commentaries are not substitutes for reading the literature itself, they will give you an idea where to go to get the real thing.

Roundsmanship '90 is divided into five sections, corresponding to the five major specialties: Internal Medicine, Surgery, Pediatrics, Obstetrics and Gynecology, and Psychiatry. Although *Roundsmanship* was originally designed for medical school students, the editors believe that every physician is and always will be a student of medicine. Read a particular section during a clinical rotation or pick it up and turn to a page at random to see what the medical world has to offer.

You will also find scattered throughout the book, Clinical Pearls. Just as on rounds, these little surprises will pop up when least expected. They range from classical wisdom passed on for ages to the latest snippet of information over a broad range of medical topics.

This book was intended for you, and we'd like to know what we can do to make it more useful. Let us know what you think about *Roundsmanship*. We'd also like for you to contribute to this book. If you have a Clinical Pearl, an original bit of medical knowledge, or a time-honored piece of medical wisdom, just mail it to us, ℅ Year Book Medical Publishers, 200 North LaSalle Street, Chicago, Illinois 60601. If it's a polished jewel, we'll publish it in the next possible edition, along with proper attribution to the sender.

Bruce B. Dan, M.D.
Editor-in-Chief

Reading and Rounds; Rounds and Reading

Ward rounds are the centerpiece of the classical pedagogic exercise of the third, and sometimes the fourth, year of medical school, the clinical clerkship. They involve, at a minimum, medical students, interns, residents, and faculty, who exchange information that is usually related to a single patient's problem. Often, specialty fellows, nurses, clinical pharmacists, and others participate as well. Rounds usually take the form of case presentations by the medical student, intern, or resident. Once the clinical problem has been placed on the table, discussion can take the form of didactic analysis of the case by the students, one of the housestaff, or, more often, the attending physician; or there may be questions and answers, or sometimes just an informal free-for-all. The location of rounds varies. They may be at the bedside, standing over the patient; sometimes in the corridor outside the patient's room, or in one of the conference rooms that exist on most floors of a teaching hospital, but the purpose of rounds has not altered in thousands of years.

However, the character of rounds has changed. In more tranquil times, they were leisurely. It was not unusual for the attending physician to spend a good deal of time with the patient, repeating the history or seeking out physical findings. I am not sure that this was the best use of the students' time, but it surely was the *modus vivendi*. More importantly, rounds were sacrosanct; few interruptions occurred or were tolerated. How times have changed! Today's rounds are both hurried and harried. Interruptions are the norm: there are phone calls and beepers that not only beep but also blare voice pages. What would Hippocrates say!

Not only is the audience constantly changing, the role of the patient on rounds has changed. A third of the time the patient is not in bed when the rounding team arrives, having been whisked off to x-ray, CT scan, ultrasound, the electrophysiology lab, and on and on. A second third of the time the patient has been discharged! When the patient is in bed there is every likelihood that a specialty fellow and/or attending is doing a history and physical. These logistic gyrations make rounding today a much more frustrating exercise for professors, housestaff, and students alike. They also make rounds much less effective than they used to be.

Although it is not a substitute for rounds, a sensible program of reading is not only necessary, it is essential. I have always believed in patient-centered reading. For students it should begin with a good current textbook—not handbooks or softcover trots. Since I have spent my life rounding in internal medicine, I refer here to one of the standard textbooks in its most current edition. The issue of currency is important; medical knowledge changes rapidly, and I cringe when I see an old edition of a textbook on the shelf. *De minimus,* the student should read the chapter dealing with the patient's illness, no matter what time of the day or night. If the library is open, he should consult one of the references that characteristically appears at the end of the chapter.

The student should make each patient a case study and approach that patient as an experiment of nature that the student is given the opportunity to observe. The student should then proceed to make a reasonably thorough search of the literature. By that I mean two or three or four of the current journals in the field—not *Deutsche Klinische Wochenschrift*. For each patient assigned to him, the student should be able to give a reasonably erudite discussion that encompasses everything from the history of the illness to the latest advances in diagnosis and therapy.

This pattern of reading should accompany each student throughout life. Since most physicians will end up taking care of patients, this pattern of reading should become a habit that can be continued.

With respect to keeping up, there are many opportunities, often at the time of examinations. In internal medicine, for example, there is the certifying examination followed a few years later by a subspecialty examination for most internists, and for a still smaller number, certificates of added competence or special qualifications. Then, in the 1990s and beyond, recertification examinations are in the offing for most of us. The type of survey reading required to pass these examinations differs from what I described above. It is more along the lines outlined by my colleague, Dr. Arnold Relman, in the 1989 edition of this book.

The thought I want to leave behind is this: Center your reading on the patient. In my experience, it makes reading more meaningful and enhances retention.

Robert G. Petersdorf
President, Association of American Medical Colleges

1
Internal Medicine

The Periodic Physical Examination in Asymptomatic Adults

Oboler SK, La Force FM
Ann Intern Med 110:214–226, Feb 1, 1989 **1–1**

Adults who are without symptoms and not pregnant do not require the traditional complete physical examination. Apart from the established screening procedures of blood pressure measurement, breast examination, and Papanicolaou (Pap) smear, it would appear useful to weigh patients, test their visual acuity and hearing, and examine their skin at appropriate intervals (Table 1). Physicians should encourage patients to have annual dental assessments. A more complete examination may be in order for those who are at increased risk because of their family history, life-style, or occupational or environmental exposure.

▸ *Here we have another look at the periodic physical examination. As shown in Table 1, our views on this subject have changed quite a bit. Three screening procedures are established: blood pressure measurement at least every 2 years, breast examination annually in women over 40, and a pelvic examination and Papanicolaou (Pap) test at least every 3 years, after 2 initial negative tests have been obtained 1 year apart. The table gives you criteria for other screening procedures.*

Trends in Cigarette Smoking in the United States: The Changing Influence of Gender and Race

Fiore MC, Novotny TE, Pierce JP, et al
JAMA 261:49–55, Jan 6, 1989 **1–2**

The impressive public health efforts made to lower the prevalence of smoking have succeeded to a degree, but the rate of decline varies with gender, race, and educational variables. A linear fall in prevalence of smoking was evident for both men and women between 1974 and 1985 (Fig 1–1). The decrease was more evident for blacks than for whites, and fewer blacks began smoking in this period. Fewer young men began smok-

TABLE 1.

Recommendations for Screening Asymptomatic Adults of Average Risk

Procedure by Age Group	Frequency
Men	
Age 20 to 59	
Blood pressure measurement	Every 2 years
Weight	Every 4 years
Dental screening	Annually
Cardiac auscultation for valve disease	Once
Skin examination for dysplastic nevi	Once
Age 60 or older	
Blood pressure measurement	Every 2 years
Weight	Every 4 years
Visual acuity	Annually
Hearing	Annually
Dental screening	Annually
Cardiac auscultation for valve disease	Once
Abdominal palpation for aortic aneurysm	Annually
Women	
Age 20 to 39	
Blood pressure measurement	Every 2 years
Weight	Every 4 years
Dental screening	Annually
Cardiac auscultation for valve disease	Once
Skin examination for dysplastic nevi	Once
Pelvic exam with Papanicolaou smear	Every 3 years†
Age 40 to 59	
Blood pressure measurement	Every 2 years
Weight	Every 4 years
Dental screening	Annually
Breast palpation*	Annually
Pelvic examination with Papanicolaou smear	Every 3 years
Age 60 or older	
Blood pressure measurement	Every 2 years
Weight	Every 4 years
Visual acuity	Annually
Hearing	Annually
Dental screening	Annually
Cardiac auscultation for valve disease	Once
Breast palpation*	Annually
Pelvic examination with Papanicolaou smear	Every 3 years

*Includes mammography.

†After 2 negative tests, 1 year apart.

(Courtesy of Oboler SK, LaForce FM: *Ann Intern Med* 110:214–226, Feb 1, 1989.)

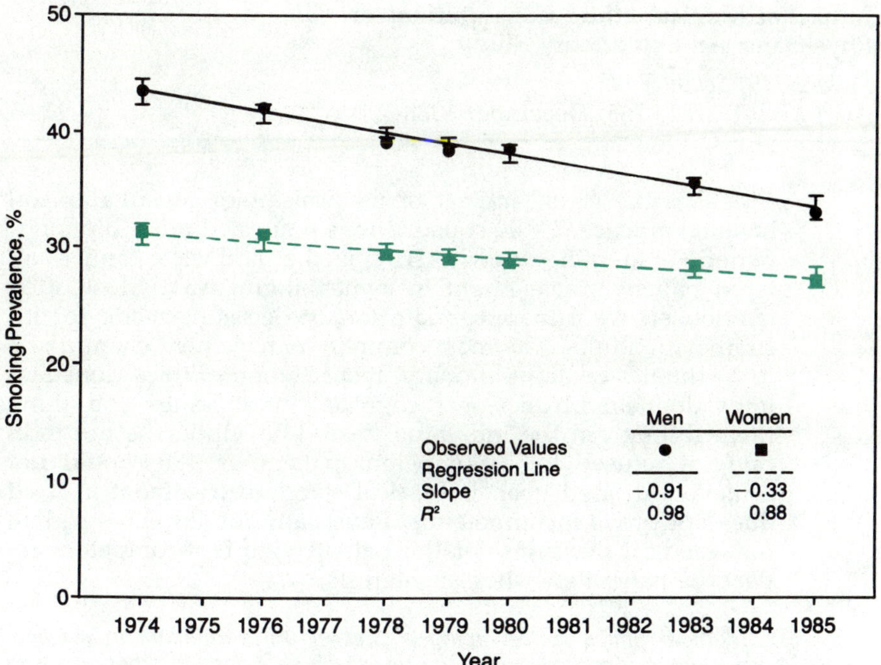

Fig 1–1
Weighted and age-standardized smoking prevalence among men and women aged 20 years and older from 1974 to 1985 in National Health Interview Surveys in the United States. (Courtesy of Fiore MC, Novotny TE, Pierce JP, et al: *JAMA* 261:49–55, Jan 6, 1989.)

ing, but young women have continued to take up smoking at the same rate as in earlier years. Updated demographic data on smoking will make it possible to identify target populations for concerted interventional efforts.

► *Cessation of smoking has become almost a fetish. I must say, as a cigar smoker, that I feel like I have lepromatous leprosy at times. Yet, one has to admit that there are unambiguous health hazards to cigarette smoking, and that the campaign of the Surgeon General and others is of value. These data show that smoking prevalence is decreasing in all race and gender groups, although the women are lagging behind.*

Impact of Medical Ethics Consultations on Physicians: An Exploratory Study

Perkins HS, Soathoff BS
Am J Med 85:761–765, December 1988 **1–3**

What is the actual impact of medical ethics consultation on hospital practice? Of 44 consultations requested in an 18-month period, 14 identified newly recognized ethical issues and 18 altered patient management in a meaningful way. Most often overlooked were inappropriate family decisions made for incompetent adults. The most common management change was to withhold cardiopulmonary resuscitation. Ethics consultations do help physicians recognize ethical issues and think them through in the individual case. Life support is not indicated if refused by a competent patient or if it would not achieve a desired goal. Refusal of standard treatment in itself does not prove incompetence. Physicians should make certain that medical decisions for the patient who is incompetent reflect the patient's wishes or interests.

▶ *Medical Ethics is becoming a part of the curriculum in medical schools and a critical part of the day-to-day activities in a hospital with desperately ill patients. Dr. Perkins from our institution summarizes his experiences in the past few years and clearly delineates the contribution that an ethics consultative service can make to clinical care.*

Estimating Physicians' Work for a Resource-Based Relative-Value Scale

Hsiao WC, Braun P, Yntema D, et al
N Engl J Med 319:835–841, Sept 29, 1988 **1–4**

Current systems of physician payment are increasingly cumbersome and complex, and they are often blamed for the increased use of medical services. An alternative system is to base reimbursement on the resource-based relative-value scale, which takes into account the total work input for each service; practice costs, including malpractice premiums; and the costs of specialty training. Estimates of physicians' work are based on time, mental effort, judgment, technical skill, physical effort, and psychological stress. A national survey of nearly 2,000 physicians in 4 specialties suggests that doctors are able to rate the relative amounts of work of the services within their specialty. The ratings are highly reproducible and probably valid. Resource-based relative values could indeed serve as a rational basis for compensating physicians.

▶ *I doubt if the surgeons would want to list this as one of their articles. It seems worthwhile to have one article such as this chosen each year. The truth of the matter is that the concept of the relative value scale may have an extraordinary effect on medical practice. I am not one who likes to make students consider economic issues, but the concepts involved in this paper are worth reading.*

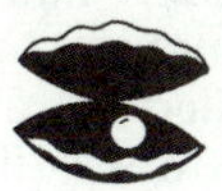

The Mercedes-Benz sign. This is a radiologic finding on KUB that is diagnostic of gallstones. It consists of stellate radiolucencies in the area of the gallbladder that appear similar to the hood ornament on a Mercedes-Benz sedan. The radiolucencies represent gas-containing fissures within the stone.

Vicissitudes of Depressed Mood During Four Years of Medical School

Clark DC, Zeldow PB
JAMA 260:2521–2528, Nov 4, 1988 **1–5**

Psychological problems in medical students often are assumed but rarely empirically assessed. This study followed a medical school class using the Beck Depression Inventory from the first day until shortly before graduation. At least 12% of the class had substantial depressive symptoms at any time during the first 3 years and 25% at the end of the second year. Individual students tended to have a constant depression ranking throughout. High scores for dysphoria did not relate to a family history of depression or to substance abuse, and women were not more vulnerable than men. Men who considered themselves to be independent and competitive were less vulnerable to dysphoria, as were women describing themselves as relatively aggressive and worldly.

▶ *What a depressing topic! I put this in to point out that psychiatrists are able to categorize and quantitate data as well. I think that each student reading this article can appreciate the problems of depression in medical school classes, housestaff training, and beyond. I think it is also important to know that this phenomenon is not related to gender.*

Selective Criteria May Increase Lumbosacral Spine Roentgenogram Use in Acute Low-Back Pain

Frazier LM, Carey TS, Lyles MF, et al
Arch Intern Med 149:47–50, January 1989 **1–6**

Among nearly 500 patients seen in 3 teaching hospital walk-in clinics with acute back pain, 1 in 5 had x-ray examinations at the initial visit. These patients tended to be older, had symptoms for a longer time, and had reflex asymmetry and point spinal tenderness. If 11 clinical criteria, compiled from expert opinion in the literature, had been applied, nearly half of the patients would have had x-ray examinations. These criteria were proposed to limit the use of lumbosacral spine radiography, but they obviously are too broad. Which criteria are truly useful remains to be learned, but nothing will replace careful clinical follow-up.

▶ *Back pain is one of the most common presenting complaints in medicine today. Thus it's amazing how little information is known about the proper way to follow a patient with this common problem, or how to examine them in the most cost-effective manner. In this study, a number of criteria were used to clarify when lumbosacral spine roentgenograms were indicated. Once again, in this era of cost containment it's important to have objective criteria and an understanding of the natural history of this common problem. I would suggest that one also read the editorial by Dr. Richard Deyo in the same issue of this journal (*Arch Intern Med *149:27, 1989).*

Multicenter Study of Autologous Adrenal Medullary Transplantation to the Corpus Striatum in Patients With Advanced Parkinson's Disease

Goetz CG, Olanow CW, Koller WC, et al
N Engl J Med 320:337–341, Feb 9, 1989 **1–7**

Nineteen patients with severe Parkinson's disease had adrenal medullary tissue transplanted to the striatum. On follow-up for 6 months, motor function improved. The proportion of "on" time without chorea more than doubled and the severity of "off" time decreased. It was not possible, however, to lower the dose of antiparkinsonian medication, and postoperative morbidity was substantial. It is premature to use this procedure widely outside research centers.

▸ *This has obviously become a very publicized and complicated issue, and it's not particularly clear whether this study puts an end to the controversy. The term that the authors use—cautious optimism—is correct, but they also emphasize that improvement is modest at best.*

Fatal Ischaemic Brain Oedema After Early Thrombolysis With Tissue Plasminogen Activator in Acute Stroke

Koudstaal PJ, Stibbe J, Vermeulen M
Br Med J 297:1571–1574, Dec 17, 1988 **1–8**

Two patients with acute major cerebral infarction involving the middle cerebral artery territory received tissue plasminogen activator, a clot-specific thrombolytic agent, within 3–4 hours after onset of symptoms. Marked fibrinogenolysis occurred, but there were no systemic bleeding complications other than bruising. Both patients deteriorated, however, and died of transtentorial herniation. The cause was not hemorrhagic transformation of the ischemic infarct, but massive cerebral edema consequent to early reperfusion. It may be that ischemia lasting for 2–5 hours damages vessels and results in leakage, whereas hemorrhage occurs only after longer periods of ischemia.

▸ *This study points out that reperfusion can be disastrous when one has underlying ischemic tissue. When a thrombolytic agent opened a thrombosed cerebral vessel, massive cerebral edema occurred. This phenomenon would be a problem mainly in a closed compartment, although the presence of free oxygen radicals during reperfusion in any tissue may cause further damage.*

Double-Masked Trial of Azathioprine in Multiple Sclerosis

British and Dutch Multiple Sclerosis Azathioprine Trial Group
Lancet 2:179–183, July 23, 1988 **1–9**

Because multiple sclerosis resembles chronic relapsing allergic encephalomyelitis, an experimental autoimmune disorder, immunosuppression has seemed worth trying. In a randomized trial of 354 patients treated with azathioprine and followed for 3 years or longer, only small differences were seen (Fig 1–2). The dosage was 2.5 mg/kg daily. The difference in relapses after 3 years was not significant, but complications did occur during azathioprine therapy. Even if there is a small benefit from azathioprine, use of this potent drug cannot be recommended for most patients. Can we find more selective and less toxic immunosuppressive treatments?

▸ *This is another example of the difficulties of the clinical trial. Here we have a disease, multiple sclerosis, that comes and goes. There is little doubt that multiple sclerosis has some resemblance to an autoimmune disease, but this is far from certain. It is a very frustrating, poorly understood entity and, unfortunately, this study just seems to further point out the problems involved. Figure 1–2 shows slight differences by 48 months in the disability status and ambulation index, but it is not clear that this warrants the use of a potent agent such as azathioprine in these patients.*

Von Hippel-Lindau Disease Affecting 43 Members of a Single Kindred

Lamiell JM, Salazar FG, Hsia YE
Medicine 68:1–29, January 1989 **1–10**

Von Hippel-Lindau disease is an inherited precancerous disorder affecting many organ systems. In this, the largest known affected kindred, there were more than 200 direct descendants in 6 generations. Half of the patients had retinal lesions and 15 had cerebellar lesions. Most had renal lesions, both cysts (Fig 1–3) and adenocarcinomas. Pancreatic cysts and epididymal masses also were frequent, but pheochromocytomas did not

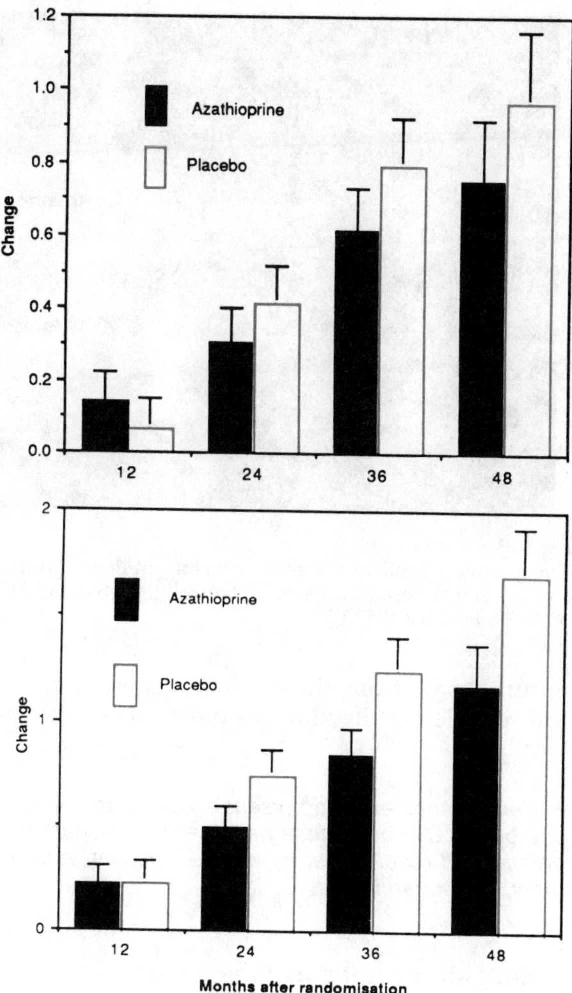

Fig 1–2
Mean changes in Kurtzke expanded disability status **(top)** and ambulation index **(bottom)** for patients taking azathioprine or placebo. *Horizontal bars,* SEM. (Courtesy of British and Dutch Multiple Sclerosis Azathioprine Trial Group: *Lancet* 2:179–183, July 23, 1988.)

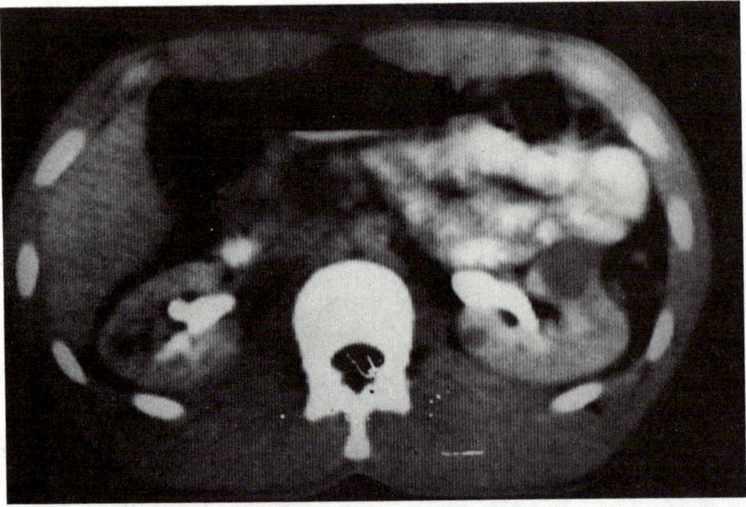

Fig 1–3
Transverse abdominal CT scan revealing multiple pancreatic and renal cysts and renal masses. (Courtesy of Lamiell JM, Salazar FG, Hsia YE: *Medicine* 68:1–29, January 1989.)

occur. Apart from these lesions there were few serious medical problems. Erythrocythemia also was absent from this family.

▶ *Here is another exotic disease that I just had to include. As you can see by the CT scan, these patients have myriad tumors, including pancreatic and renal cysts, as well as vascular and renal tumors, among them, adenocarcinoma.*

The Non-Hodgkin Lymphoma Pathologic Classification Project: Long-Term Follow-Up of 1153 Patients With Non-Hodgkin Lymphomas

Simon R, Durrleman S, Hoppe RT, et al
Ann Intern Med 109:939–945, Dec 15, 1988 **1–11**

Patients at 3 referral centers in the United States and 1 in Italy were followed for a median of 11 years. More than two thirds had died by the time of analysis. Patients with lymphomas of low, intermediate, and high grade had respective 10-year survival rates of 45%, 26%, and 23%. Intermediate- and high-grade lymphomas were curable, but advanced-stage, low-grade lesions were not. The Ann Arbor staging system made a prognostic distinction between patients with stage I and those with more extensive low-grade follicular lymphomas. The system also predicted survival according to stage for patients having diffuse large cell and immunoblastic lymphomas.

▶ *The non-Hodgkin's lymphomas are a diverse group of conditions. Oncologists are great at forming various classification systems, and I gave up on this a long time ago. This study, however, seems to simplify the nomenclature, and I would refer the student to the original article for more details.*

A Randomized Clinical Trial Evaluating Sequential Methotrexate and Fluorouracil in the Treatment of Patients With Node-Negative Breast Cancer Who Have Estrogen-Receptor-Negative Tumors

Fisher B, Redmond C, Dimitrov NV, et al
N Engl J Med 320:473–478, Feb 23, 1989 **1–12**

Is sequential methotrexate-fluorouracil-leucovorin therapy worthwhile in women with breast cancers lacking estrogen receptor whose axillary nodes are negative? In a series of nearly 700 such patients, disease-free survival was significantly better in treated patients of all ages (Fig 1–4). After 4 years, treatment failures were halved in patients aged 50 or more. Local, regional, and distant disease all were controlled to some degree and side effects were tolerable. This regimen is suitable for women who choose not to participate in clinical trials. It also could be used in the control arm of trials done to assess new treatments.

▶ *This article is 1 of 4 separate critical papers on therapy of patients with breast cancer who were node negative at the time of initial treatment. There are also editorials by McGuire and by DeVita, in the same issue of this journal (pp 525 and 527). In essence, all of these studies found improvement in disease-free survival, but after follow-up periods of 3–5 years there was no clear-cut improvement in overall survival. Breast cancer is a complicated disease, especially in node-negative patients, and I would refer each of you to this issue of the* New England Journal of Medicine *to develop your own perspective.*

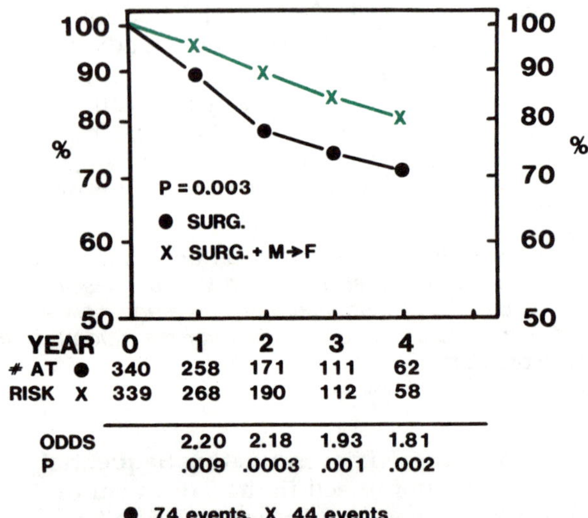

Fig 1–4
Disease-free survival according to treatment group. *Crosses,* percentages of patients surviving in the group treated with sequential methotrexate and fluorouracil as adjuvant therapy; *solid circles,* values in the group treated with surgery alone. "Events" included deaths not caused by cancer, recurrences of breast cancer, or occurrences of a second tumor. (Courtesy of Fisher B, Redmond C, Dimitrov NV, et al: *N Engl J Med* 320:473–478, Feb 23, 1989.)

First Results on Mortality Reduction in the UK Trial of Early Detection of Breast Cancer

UK Trial of Early Detection of Breast Cancer Group
Lancet 2:411–416, Aug 20, 1988 **1–13**

In the UK trial almost 46,000 women 45–64 years of age had annual clinical examination of the breasts and mammography in alternate years. Another 63,000 women were offered instruction in breast self-examination. Population-adjusted breast cancer mortality was 14% lower in screened women over a 7-year period, but the difference is not yet statistically significant. Importantly, the effect of screening is increasingly apparent after the first 5 years (Fig 1–5). Breast self-examination alone has not lowered the death rate in breast cancer.

▶ *There is a lot of controversy about the various screening procedures. This paper reports an extensive study and would seem to indicate that there is a substantial reduction in mortality from breast cancer with*

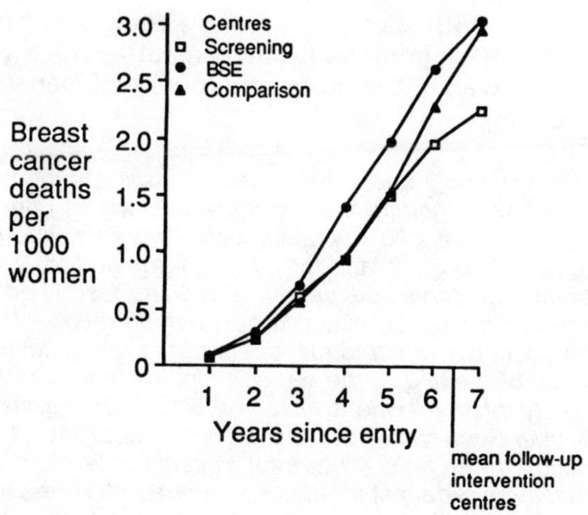

Fig 1–5
Cumulative breast cancer mortality rate per 1,000 women in screening centers, breast self-examination centers, and comparison centers in successive years after entry into trial. (Courtesy of UK Trial of Early Detection of Breast Cancer Group: *Lancet* 2:411–416, Aug 20, 1988.)

early detection. The economists seem to have a lot of fun evaluating the number of diagnoses per $100,000 spent in screening and other types of parameters, and it becomes a complex issue of the finances of health care delivery.

Role of Sigmoidoscopy in Screening for Colorectal Cancer: A Critical Review

Neugut AI, Pita S
Gastroenterology 95:492–499, August 1988 **1–14**

It seems that screening for occult fecal blood has generated more controversy than sigmoidoscopy in detecting colorectal cancers. No randomized controlled trial has specifically addressed the role of endoscopy in screening for colon cancer. One that comes close, a Kaiser Foundation study enrolling more than 5,000 persons, provides the best evidence available that sigmoidoscopic screening is effective; deaths caused by "potentially postponable" causes were 30% fewer in the study group. But this is not the last word. Those at increased risk of colorectal cancer such as close relatives of cancer patients and persons with ulcerative colitis should be individually considered. For asymptomatic persons at average risk the physician has to weigh the costs and potential benefits of endoscopic screening.

▶ *The periodic health examination is still a controversial topic. At one time it was thought that an individual would come to a fancy clinic, have a massive "blue plate special" work-up, and that this was an extremely important and well-proven method of preventive medicine. When one studies the various screening tests, however, there are only a few that have an effective cost-benefit ratio. This paper reviews sigmoidoscopy, which to me is one of the few potential screening procedures of merit. Yet, the paper indicates that even this test is not completely proven. One should remember, however, that the American Cancer Society includes 3 screening modalities: (1) digital rectal examination on an annual basis for patients older than 40 years; (2) an annual stool slide test for those older than 50 years; and (3) a sigmoidoscopy every 3–5 years after 2 initial negative examinations, 1 year apart, for persons older than 50 years. Also, you should review a previous paper concerning this issue (see Abstract 1–1).*

Common Inheritance of Susceptibility to Colonic Adenomatous Polyps and Associated Colorectal Cancers

Cannon-Albright LA, Skolnick MH, Bishop DT, et al
N Engl J Med 319:533–537, Sept 1, 1988 **1–15**

Nearly 700 members of 34 Utah kindreds underwent proctosigmoidoscopy to 60 cm. Either a single proband had an adenomatous polyp or a cluster of relatives had colorectal cancer. Adenomas were discovered in 19% of the relatives of probands and in 12% of spouses. The most likely genetic model is that adenomatous polyps and colorectal cancers occur only in genetically susceptible persons. Inherited susceptibility probably accounts for most clinical colonic neoplasms. At the same time, environmental factors, particularly diet, are important. Screening is in order for first-degree relatives of persons having either colorectal cancer or adenomatous polyps.

▶ *This study confirms and extends previous observations of a group having inherited susceptibility to adenomatous polyps and colorectal cancer. Previously, the authors had studied a single kindred; now they have added 33 additional families. The studies indicated that screening protocols should be modified when there is a genetic predisposition to colonic neoplasia. This is just one of a number of important genetic studies that have been done in large families in Utah.*

Effect of Recombinant Human Granulocyte-Macrophage Colony-Stimulating Factor on Chemotherapy-Induced Myelosuppression

Antman KS, Griffin JD, Elias A, et al
N Engl J Med 319:593–598, Sept 8, 1988 **1–16**

Myelosuppression often limits chemotherapy for cancer. In the hope of countering this effect, 16 adults with inoperable or metastatic sarcoma received increasing doses of recombinant human granulocyte-macrophage colony-stimulating factor (rhGM-CSF) at the time of a first cycle of chemotherapy. The white blood cell count rose substantially (Fig 1–6), and neutropenia was significantly less severe and lasted for a shorter time than in a second cycle of therapy when rhGM-CSF was not given. Doses of more than 32 μg/kg daily produced edema and thrombosis. This is a promising adjunct to cancer chemotherapy, but whether infectious morbidity is lowered remains to be seen.

▶ *Another chapter in the use of rhGM-CSF in patients with malignancies. The agents cause only mild side effects and are highly active in leukopenic patients. We will just have to get more information before we know how useful these compounds can be, but they do have tremendous potential.*

Clinical Significance of a Single Test for Anti-Cardiolipin Antibodies in Patients With Systemic Lupus Erythematosus

Kalunian KC, Peter JB, Middlekauff HR, et al
Am J Med 85:602–608, November 1988 **1–17**

What is the true significance of anticardiolipin antibodies (aCL) in patients with systemic lupus? An enzyme-linked immunosorbent assay was used in 85 consecutive outpatients with systemic lupus and 40 controls in seeking an answer to this question. Antibody was present in more than 40% of the lupus patients and in 7.5% of controls. In the patients, aCL correlated with thrombosis, thrombocytopenia, and fetal loss, but

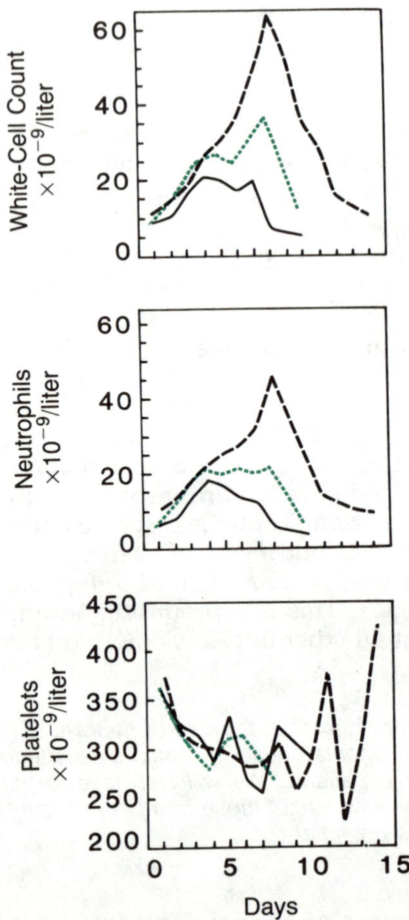

Fig 1–6
Mean of total daily leukocyte, neutrophil, and platelet counts during cycle 0 before chemotherapy according to dose level of rhGM-CSF. *Solid line,* 6 patients who received a 4-μg or 8-μg dose of rhGM-CSF per kg daily; *dotted line,* 6 patients who received 16-μg or 32-μg doses; *dashed line,* 4 patients who received a 64-μg dose. (Courtesy of Antman KS, Griffin JD, Elias A, et al: *N Engl J Med* 319:593–598, Sept 8, 1988.)

not with disease activity or severity. The test has 2 obvious applications: in lupus patients considering pregnancy, and in those with a history of thrombosis.

► *There are so many antibodies that have been delineated in patients with various collagen diseases that it does get confusing. On the other hand, the aCLs seen in some patients with lupus are especially intriguing. There is an association between this antibody and various thrombotic events, thrombocytopenia, and fetal loss. In the lupus patient who becomes pregnant, you must perform the aCL test.*

Clinical and Immunologic Effects of Monthly Administration of Intravenous Cyclophosphamide in Severe Systemic Lupus Erythematosus

McCune WJ, Gobbus J, Zeldes W, et al
N Engl J Med 318:1423–1431, June 2, 1988 **1–18**

Steroids may fail to save patients who have severe systemic lupus involving the kidneys or central nervous system. Nine such patients, refractory to oral steroids, received monthly intravenous infusions of cyclophosphamide for half a year; the initial dose was 500 mg/m^2. Central nervous system symptoms

TABLE 2.
Clinical Changes in Patients Treated With Intravenous Cyclophosphamide

Variable	Pretreatment	Follow-up†	P Value
24-hour urinary protein (g)	4.11±1.2	0.90±0.34	<0.05
Creatinine clearance (ml/min)	0.64±0.8 ml/sec/m^2	0.93±0.9 ml/sec/m^2	<0.001
Serum creatinine (μmol/liter)	124±18	115±18	NS
Westergren ESR (mm/hr)	60.2±9.8	34.4±8.7	<0.0005
Anti-DNA (% binding)	43±11	8.5±1.6	<0.01
Total complement (CH_{50} units)	88.7±14.7	113.4±9.7	<0.05
Complement C3 (mg/liter)	894±145	1150±83	<0.05
Complement C4 (mg/liter)	154±28	222±38	<0.05
Prednisone dosage (mg/day)	45±5.2	17±2.8	<0.01

To convert values for creatinine clearance to mL/minute, multiply by 103. To convert values for serum creatinine to mg/dL, multiply by 0.01131. Plus–minus values are means ±SEM; *NS*, not significant; *ESR*, erythrocyte sedimentation rate.

†Approximately 6 weeks after treatment.

(Courtesy of McCune WJ, Golbus J, Zeldes W, et al: *N Engl J Med* 318:1423–1431, June 2, 1988.)

resolved in 3 patients, but in another patient new features of disease developed during treatment. Renal function improved substantially, along with many laboratory parameters of the disease (Table 2). The T lymphocytes subsets remained lowered after treatment.

▶ *You name a therapeutic agent and it's been used in the treatment of systemic lupus, here a monthly intravenous infusion of cyclophosphamide for 6 months. The results are very encouraging and indicate both clinical and immunologic regression of the disease. As the authors state at the end, the study was "a preliminary, uncontrolled study, but the results warrant further investigation of this form of treatment." We certainly hope that further studies confirm these good results. I was especially impressed with the 50% improvement in renal function and the 80% reduction in urinary protein excretion.*

The Effect of Dietary Supplementation With n-3 Polyunsaturated Fatty Acids on the Synthesis of Interleukin-1 and Tumor Necrosis Factor by Mononuclear Cells

Endres S, Ghorbani R, Kelley VE, et al
N Engl J Med 320:265–271, Feb 2, 1989 **1–19**

Patients with rheumatoid disease and psoriasis have benefited clinically from dietary supplementation with n-3 fatty acids. The explanation might lie in lowered production of interleukin-1 and tumor necrosis factor, the chief polypeptide mediators of inflammation. Impaired production of both factors was indeed confirmed when 9 healthy volunteers added fish oil concentrate to their diets for 6 weeks and factor synthesis by endotoxin-stimulated blood mononuclear cells was examined in vitro. An intriguing question: Do other unsaturated fatty acids have similar effects?

▶ *Interleukin-1 and tumor necrosis factor are the principal polypeptide mediators of inflammation. Thus reduction in production of these cytokines might contribute to amelioration of inflammatory symptoms. This interesting paper suggests that administration of long-chain n-3 fatty acids caused a marked decrease in production of these substances. This is very important information, and we await further studies to delineate the clinical significance.*

Diagnostic Radionuclide Imaging of Amyloid: Biological Targeting by Circulating Human Serum Amyloid P Component

Hawkins PN, Myers MJ, Lavender JP, et al
Lancet 1:1413–1418, June 25, 1988 **1–20**

If systemic amyloidosis could be diagnosed early, aggressive anti-inflammatory treatment might halt or even reverse the process. An imaging technique was developed that uses ^{123}I-labeled purified human serum amyloid P (SAP) component, which has affinity for all types of amyloid fibrils. In 14 patients with various types of amyloid disease, specific uptake into amyloid deposits was observed; in 5 controls there was no tissue localization of the label. Once sequestered in amyloid deposits the activity persisted for a long time. If SAP can be coupled to an agent that destroys amyloid fibrils, a promising therapeutic approach might be at hand.

▶ *I am fascinated by amyloidosis. It seems always to be the obscure diagnosis in a clinicopathologic conference in the* New England Journal of Medicine. *When I was a medical student, one talked about staining tissue with Congo red or whatever, but here we have a diagnosis being made with quantitation of the localization of amyloid with labeled light chain components. It seems to be applicable to several forms of the disease, and one could clearly begin to think ahead to therapeutic maneuvers as well. This is truly an exciting paper.*

Screening for Diabetes Mellitus

Singer DE, Samet JH, Coley CM, et al
Ann Intern Med 109:639–649, Oct 15, 1988 **1–21**

Screening for diabetes (Table 3) makes sense only when starting treatment before symptoms develop is more effective than later. But even then, screening might not be appropriate: Less than accurate screening, and dangerous or unduly expensive procedures, can make these programs more costly in both health and dollar terms than they are worth. Screening for gestational diabetes may be useful because it is not costly and there is a real, although small, expected benefit. On the other hand, screening of nonpregnant adults is not recommended. The link between better glucose control and a lower risk of diabetic complications remains weak. This is not to say that cer-

TABLE 3.
Recommendations for Screening for Diabetes Mellitus

Type of Diabetes	Possible Rationale for Screening	Recommendation
Gestational	Gestational diabetes has been associated with pregnancy loss and complications. Glycemic control appears to improve outcome. Gestational diabetes may be silent.	Screening for gestational diabetes may be beneficial and is not likely to incur much risk or cost. Screening of all pregnant women seems reasonable. The screening test should be a 50-g glucose load given between weeks 24 and 28. Patients with plasma glucose values greater than 140 mg/dL at 1 hour should have a full oral glucose tolerance test.
Pregestational (women planning to become pregnant)	Diabetic patients who become pregnant face substantial risks for pregnancy loss and other complications. Careful glycemic control and obstetric management reduces these risks.	"Silent" diabetes of child-bearing age is probably rare. The pregnancy risk faced by such women and the benefits of early therapy are not known. Screening of women at heightened risk for diabetes may be reasonable, but there is little evidence bearing on this issue.

Type I	Early therapy may forestall complications. Immunosuppressive therapy may prevent further beta-cell destruction.	The prevalence of type I diabetes detectable by screening is small. The benefits of early hypoglycemic therapy are unknown. Immunosuppressive strategies are still experimental. Screening is not currently recommended.
Type II	The prevalence of undiagnosed impaired glucose tolerance or type II diabetes is substantial. Early intervention might prevent deterioration of impaired glucose tolerance to frank diabetes, or improve glycemic control among diabetic patients and thereby prevent vascular and neurologic complications. Identification of undiagnosed diabetic patients might lead to early diagnosis of vision-threatening retinopathy and timely laser therapy.	The benefits of early diagnosis and therapy in preventing worsening glucose tolerance or diabetic complications have not been shown. Vision-threatening retinopathy rarely precedes the diagnosis of diabetes. Screening for type II diabetes is not recommended. For selected obese persons, screening for impaired glucose tolerance or diabetes may better motivate weight loss, which may prevent progression of glucose intolerance.

(Courtesy of Singer DE, Samet JH, Coley CM, et al: *Ann Intern Med* 109:639–649, Oct 15, 1988.)

tain patients would not benefit from screening. An example: the obese patient who would be willing to lose weight if glucose intolerance is demonstrated.

► *I know that everyone hears about the importance of screening for diabetes, but I think that this article from the group at Massachusetts General does indeed put a damper on that thought. Their current recommendation is that screening is useful only in gestational diabetes. Obviously, as our knowledge of the use of immunosuppressive therapy for early type I diabetes expands, this advice may change. I recommend reading this entire article.*

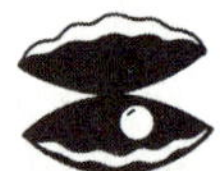

Generalized exfoliative dermatitis—think of 3 causes: drug hypersensitivity, preexisting skin disease such as psoriasis, and *lymphoma.*

Factors Associated With Early Remission of Type I Diabetes in Children Treated With Cyclosporine

Bougneres PF, Carel JC, Castano L, et al
N Engl J Med 318:663–670, March 17, 1988 **1–22**

If, as seems increasingly certain, type I insulin-dependent diabetes is of autoimmune origin, immunosuppressive treatment is logical. In a pilot study of 40 children with recently diagnosed diabetes, 27 were able to stop using insulin when given daily cyclosporine therapy. After a full year, half of the patients still did not require insulin. Trough drug levels were kept at 150–350 ng/mL. Patients who had lost the least amount of weight were the most likely to have remission. Another predictor of response was a higher C-peptide level on initial glucagon testing. The immunosuppressive approach is grounded on detecting hyperglycemia early in those with genetic and immunologic markers of type I diabetes.

► *I still have a hard time getting used to the idea that juvenile-onset diabetes or insulin-dependent diabetes, whatever name you want to use, is frequently an immunologic disorder; yet, the evidence now is incontrovertible. Here we have the logical follow-up for this: another clinical trial evaluating the use of agents such as cyclosporine in children with recent-onset type I diabetes. The results are fairly good, and this may become standard therapy one day. Not yet, however.*

Impaired Pulsatile Secretion of Insulin in Relatives of Patients With Non-Insulin-Dependent Diabetes

O'Rahily S, Turner RC, Matthews DR
N Engl J Med 318:1225–1230, May 12, 1988 **1–23**

Normal persons secrete regular pulses of insulin every 12–15 minutes, but patients with non-insulin-dependent diabetes do not. Ten first-degree relatives of patients whose glucose tolerance was not very abnormal had higher fasting plasma glucose levels than controls had. They lacked regular oscillatory activ-

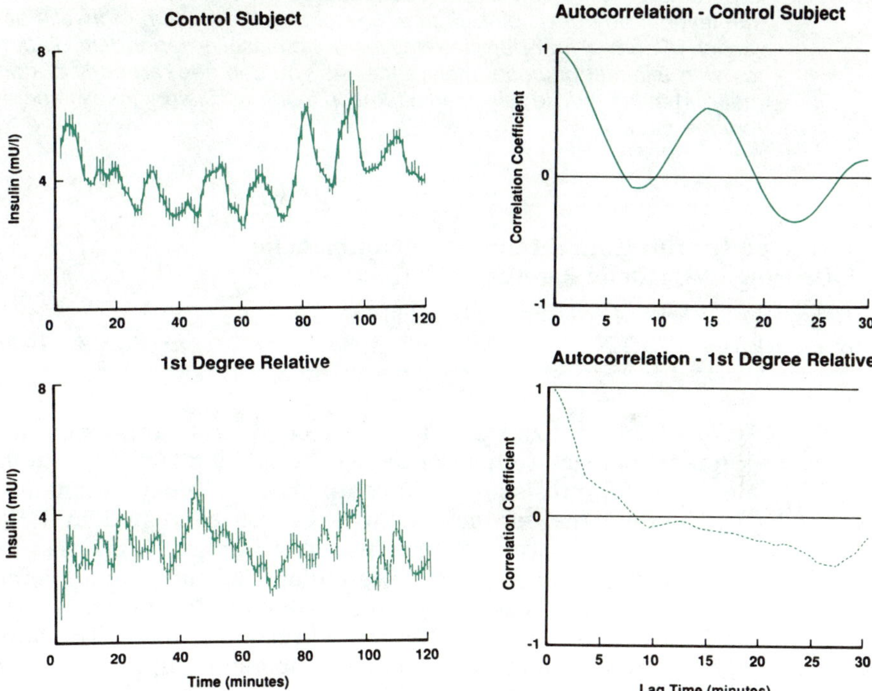

Fig 1–7
Stationarized plasma insulin profile and autocorrelogram of a relative of a patient with non-insulin-dependent diabetes and of a control. **Top 2 panels,** plasma insulin profile of a 3-point moving average (±SEM) of 1-minute samples obtained in a period of 150 minutes in a control and a relative. The control had regular insulin pulses every 12–15 minutes; the relative did not. **Bottom 2 panels,** autocorrelograms of the basal plasma insulin data on the same persons. The control had a significant negative-to-positive peak at 12–14 minutes; the relative did not. (Courtesy of O'Rahily S, Turner RC, Matthews DR, et al: *N Engl J Med* 318:1225–1230, May 12, 1988.)

ity, and no significant peak was apparent (Fig 1–7). The insulin secretory response to intravenous glucose was unimpaired. Pulsatile insulin secretion may help to maintain target tissue sensitivity, and impaired oscillatory secretion may be an early event in the development of non-insulin-dependent diabetes.

▶ *There once was a time when an individual could study insulin release just by taking a plasma sample and measuring the immunoreactive blood level. Now we've learned much more. We must recognize that this is an oscillating secretory mechanism, and that it is almost as important to delineate the time sequence as it is to determine the absolute level at any one point. Figure 1–7 shows the pattern of insulin secretion in normal first-degree relatives of non-insulin-dependent diabetics with minimal glucose intolerance. As you can see, an early abnormality in these individuals is an alteration in the oscillatory insulin secretory mechanism.*

Increased Insulin Concentrations in Nondiabetic Offspring of Diabetic Parents

Haffner SM, Stern MP, Hazuda HP, et al
N Engl J Med 319:1297–1301, Nov 17, 1988 **1–24**

It was hypothesized that the elevated risk of non-insulin-dependent diabetes (NIDDM) caused by genetic factors is mediated by insulin resistance and compensatory hyperinsulinemia. To test this, the serum insulin level was estimated in 1,500 nondiabetic Mexican Americans, a group at high risk of NIDDM. If 1 or both parents were diabetic, the fasting insulin level increased accordingly, even after controlling for body mass index, body fat distribution, and blood glucose. The finding of hyperinsulinemia in prediabetic persons supports insulin resistance as a cause of NIDDM.

▶ *I believe that this is a very important epidemiologic study, using the Hispanic population of San Antonio. Diabetes mellitus is an extraordinarily common problem in our population, and Haffner and associates have examined this entity in great detail. This particular paper clearly indicates that prediabetic individuals have hyperinsulinemia. The results suggest that, in one way or another, insulin resistance plays a role in at least the early phases of hyperinsulinemia.*

Glucose Control and the Renal and Retinal Complications of Insulin-Dependent Diabetes

Chase HP, Jackson WE, Hoops SL, et al
JAMA 261:1155–1160, Feb 24, 1989 **1–25**

This study looks into how closely glucose control relates to diabetic complications. In 230 insulin-dependent diabetics, serious retinopathy was more than twice as frequent in those with long-term poor control (Fig 1–8) and microalbuminuria was more than 3 times as frequent. When the mean glycohemoglobin value remained consistently within 1.1 times the upper normal limit, retinopathy and albuminuria were not seen. The duration of diabetes contributed to both risks, and age was a factor in the development of retinopathy.

▶ *One of the many controversial areas in medicine today is the relationship between diabetic control and the development of complications. This is one of a massive number of papers addressing this issue*

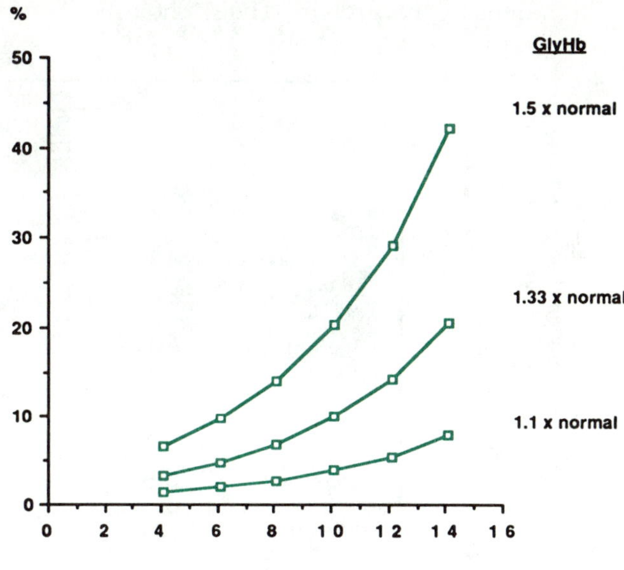

Fig 1–8
Risk of having level 3–6 retinopathy by age 15 years for given mean glycohemoglobin level (for all values ever done) and for duration of diabetes. *Normal* refers to upper limit of normal (8.2%). (Courtesy of Chase HP, Jackson WE, Hoops SL, et al: *JAMA* 261:1155–1160, Feb 24, 1989.)

and, as shown in Figure 1–8, the risk for severe diabetic retinopathy developing is directly related to evaluation of the glycohemoglobin concentration. These studies indicate that the tighter the control, the lower the incidence of complications. This is a tricky subject and one that is still far from settled.

Changes in Plasma Lipids and Lipoproteins in Overweight Men During Weight Loss Through Dieting as Compared With Exercise

Wood PD, Stefanick ML, Dreon DM, et al
N Engl J Med 319:1173–1179, Nov 3, 1988 **1–26**

Given only one way of normalizing the plasma lipids and lipoproteins, is diet or exercise better? This question was addressed in a well-publicized trial of 155 sedentary overweight men aged 30–59 years who had basically normal treadmill tests. Both the dieters and those who exercised, chiefly by running, lost total body weight and fat weight. The plasma level of high-density lipoprotein (HDL) cholesterol increased in both

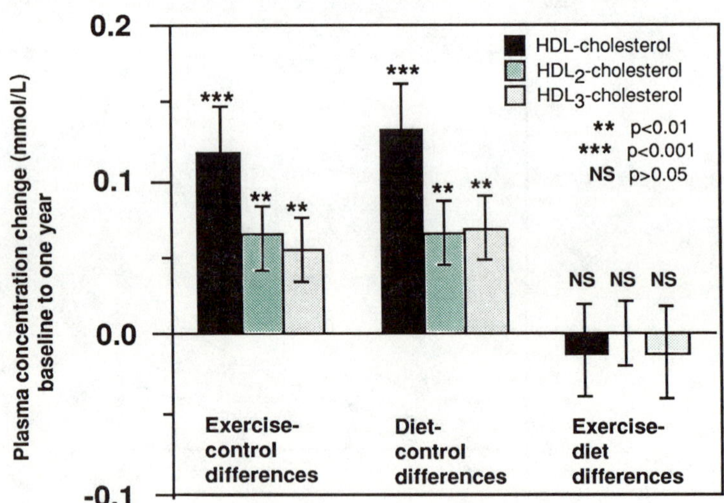

Fig 1–9
Differences between the 1-year changes in plasma concentrations of HDL cholesterol, HDL_2 cholesterol, and HDL_3 cholesterol in the study groups. *NS*, not significant. Values are the difference between the differences in the exercise and diet groups and the control group. (Courtesy of Wood PD, Stefanick ML, Dreon DM, et al: *N Engl J Med* 319:1173–1179, Nov 3, 1988.)

groups (Fig 1–9), and triglycerides fell significantly. However, the level of low-density lipoprotein cholesterol did not change significantly with either regimen. Apparently, body fat loss, whether from diet or increased exercise, produces favorable changes in HDL cholesterol and its subfractions.

► *This study hit the front pages of virtually every newspaper. As shown in Figure 1–9, there really are no differences in the changes in various lipid parameters with exercise or diet. The thing I am worried about is what happens to those individuals who don't like to exercise and love to eat. I guess we have a problem.*

The Natural History of Untreated Hyperprolactinemia: A Prospective Analysis

Schlechte J, Dolan K, Sherman B, et al
J Clin Endocrinol Metab 68:412–418, February 1989 **1–27**

What happens to hyperprolactinemic women if they are merely followed up? It is possible that treatment will rarely be necessary. One third of a group of 30 such women improved symptomatically and had declining hormone levels. Those who were amenorrheic, however, usually did not improve (Fig 1–10, p 28). Six women in the study had increased serum prolactin levels. In 4 women evidence of pituitary tumor developed during the study, but none had a macroadenoma or pituitary hypofunction. Even readily identified prolactinomas have a limited growth potential.

► *Hyperprolactinemia is a common endocrinologic problem. This prospective study from the University of Iowa indicates that the natural history is not one of progression. In fact, without any therapy, many of these patients have clinical and radiographic improvement.*

Transsphenoidal Microsurgery for Cushing Disease: A Report of 216 Cases

Mampalam TJ, Tyrrell JB, Wilson CB
Ann Intern Med 109:487–493, Sept 15, 1988 **1–28**

Surgical candidates in this series were selected on endocrinologic grounds with the aid of magnetic resonance imaging and selective venous sampling for ACTH. Cushing's disease remit-

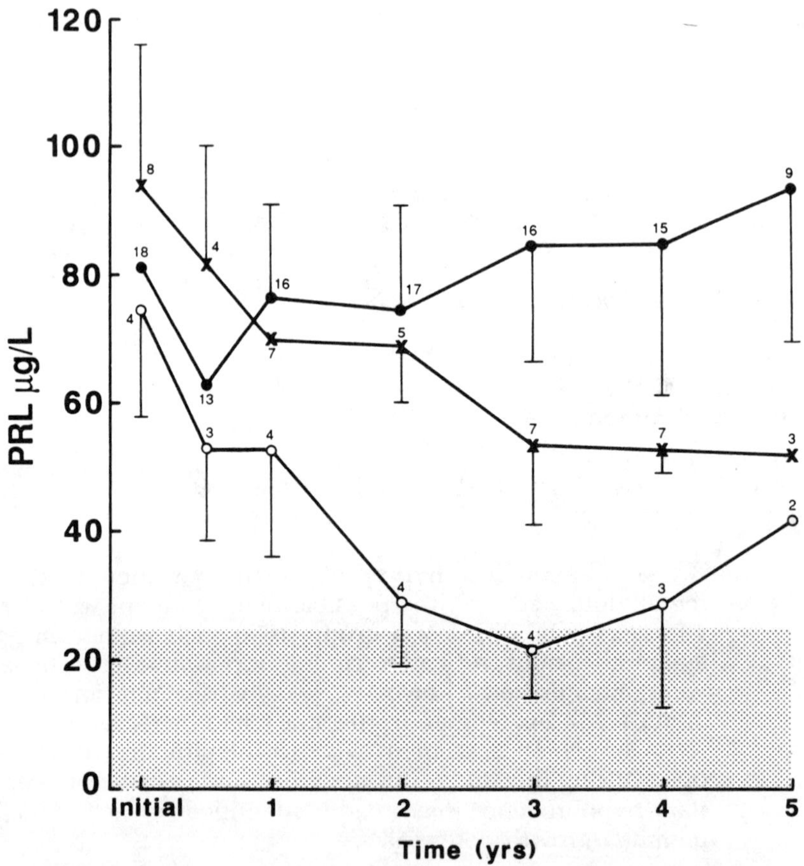

Fig 1–10
Mean (±SE) serum prolactin (PRL) levels at the initial visit and at yearly intervals in hyperprolactinemic women with amenorrhea *(filled circles)*, oligomenorrhea **(X)**, or regular menstrual periods *(open circles)*. *Numbers,* patients studied at each time point; *Shaded area,* normal range for serum PRL. (Courtesy of Schlechte J, Dolan K, Sherman B, et al: *J Clin Endocrinol Metab* 68:412–418, February 1989.)

ted in 76% of the group. Remission was most likely when an adenoma was confirmed histologically, in cases of microadenoma, and when disease was limited to the sella. About 10% of patients had complictions, but there were no deaths directly related to transsphenoidal surgery. This approach can be recommended for most patients with Cushing's disease. Extracellular extension is the chief determinant of the outcome.

▶ *This is a fine clinical review. Selective transsphenoidal adenomectomy is without doubt the primary treatment now for most patients with Cushing's disease. The procedure seems preferable to bilateral adrenalectomy, pituitary radiation, total hypophysectomy, or administration of any type of drug therapy. The complication rate is low and the success rate high. Harvey Cushing would be quite pleased.*

Overnight Clonidine Suppression Test in the Diagnosis and Exclusion of Pheochromocytoma

MacDougall IC, Isles CG, Stewart H, et al
Am J Med 84:993–1000, June 1988 **1–29**

Here is a new entry in the seemingly endless quest for the perfect way of diagnosing pheochromocytoma. The overnight test with 0.3 mg of clonidine identified 12 patients with pheochromocytoma from among 19 suspect hypertensive patients without this lesion and 31 other hypertensive patients not suspected to have pheochromocytoma (Fig 1–11, p 30). Four patients with pheochromocytoma had equivocal plasma catecholamine levels. The combination of clonidine and sleep suppressed urinary levels of catecholamines to less than 20 nmol/mmol of creatinine.

▶ *This is a nice detailed study of the "zillionth" method of diagnosing pheochromocytoma. In fact, there are probably as many ways to diagnose the disease as there are patients. Seriously, this is a logical, safe test that might be of value in certain situations, such as when there is only an equivocal elevation of plasma catecholamine levels.*

Anabolic Steroids: The Power and the Glory?

Ferner RE, Rawlins MD
Br Med J 297:877–878, Oct 8, 1988 **1–30**

Ben Johnson, disqualified in the recent Olympics, is only a recent and prominent example of an accomplished athlete using anabolic steroids in a wish to be first and best. It is far from certain that anabolic androgens improve athletic performance more than diet and training alone. Most double-blind trials have failed to show convincing change in standard tests of strength. Claims that athletes are not susceptible to the toxic effects of these drugs are easily refuted. Among these, one may

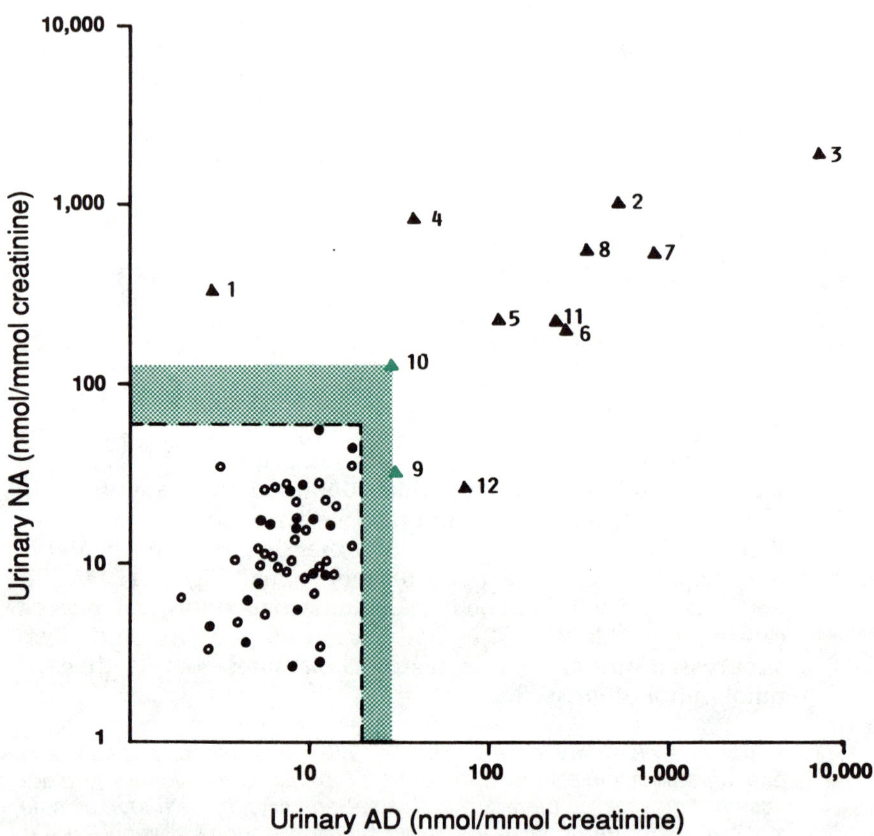

Fig 1–11
Urinary levels of norepinephrine (NA) and epinephrine (AD) during sleep after clonidine administration in 62 patients. *Dotted line,* the highest values recorded in patients who did not have pheochromocytoma. The *shaded area* indicates that there was no overlap between the data of controls and of patients with pheochromocytoma, all of whom were identified correctly using this test. *Triangles,* patients with pheochromocytoma; *open circles,* patients in whom pheochromocytoma was suspected but later excluded; *filled circles,* patients in whom pheochromocytoma was never suspected. (Courtesy of MacDougall IC, Isles CG, Stewart H, et al: *Am J Med* 84:993–1000, June 1988.)

count liver dysfunction, insulin resistance, increased blood pressure, hypercholesterolemia, myocardial infarction, and psychosis. The added threats of hypogonadism and gynecomastia might dissuade even a committed athlete from using anabolic steroids. Even if an athlete is convinced of the efficacy of anabolic steroids, this grim list of possible side effects should give pause.

▶ *I know that everyone thinks that medical journals are boring, sedate, and uninteresting. The original article includes a picture of Ben Johnson beating Carl Lewis in the recent olympics. The article points out that in 1889 Brown Sequard, a famous name in medicine, attempted to restore his failing powers with injections of an extract of crushed guinea pig testicles. Very few concepts are new.*

Abnormal Red-Cell Calcium Pump in Patients With Idiopathic Hypercalciuria

Bianchi G, Vezzoli G, Cusi D, et al
N Engl J Med 319:897–901, Oct 6, 1988 **1–31**

The genetic features of idiopathic hypercalciuria, which often underlies calcium nephrolithiasis, suggest a defect in some enzyme activity involved in calcium transport across cell membranes. An obvious candidate is calcium-magnesium-ATPase. Thirty-eight patients with a history of calcium oxalate stones had increased red cell-membrane enzyme activity as well as increased sodium-potassium pump activity. In renal stone patients with either increased or normal calcium excretion, calcium-magnesium-ATPase activity correlated well with 24-hour urinary calcium excretion.

▶ *Idiopathic hypercalcuria is the abnormality associated most frequently with renal stones. Several pathogenetic subtypes have been proposed, including increased gastrointestinal absorption, a renal calcium transport abnormality, altered bone reabsorption, and alterations in the regulation of 1,25 dyhydroxy-vitamin D_3 synthesis. This intriguing paper from the University of Milan suggests a generalized transport defect in calcium magnesium ATPase.*

Local and Systemic Factors in the Pathogenesis of Osteoporosis

Raisz LG
N Engl J Med 318:818–828, March 31, 1988 **1–32**

Osteoporosis, a decrease in bone mass and strength, entails a reduction in the number of trabecular bone plates and conversion of the plates to rods. The structure is weakened more than might be expected from the absolute decline in bone mass. Apart from calcium-regulating and growth-regulating hormones and sex hormones, osteoporosis may reflect abnormalities in local factors influencing bone cell function such as prostaglandins, interleukins, and osteoclast-activating factors. Some osteoporotic patients may have structural changes in collagen, which provides the bulk of the bone matrix. Treatments based on reversing obvious contributory factors (such as immobilization and reduced calcium intake) have had limited success. More rational measures will become available if specific disease mechanisms can be identified.

▶ *Osteoporosis has emerged as one of the major health problems in the United States. Fortunately, the science delineating the basis for this disease has progressed commensurately. Many laboratories are working on the development of new agents that indeed may impede bone loss, and I think this is one of the most exciting areas in all of internal medicine today.*

Hungry Bone Syndrome: Clinical and Biochemical Predictors of Its Occurrence After Parathyroid Surgery

Brasier AR, Nussbaum SR
Am J Med 84:654–660, April 1988 **1–33**

Extensive remineralization of the skeleton after surgery for primary hyperparathyroidism can lead to persistent hypocalcemia, hypophosphatemia, and even tetany. Albright called this the "hungry bone syndrome." Affected patients need intensive calcium and vitamin D supplementation for a long time. Twenty-five of 218 patients admitted for surgery for primary hyperparathyroidism had the hungry bone syndrome. They were older than the other patients and had higher baseline calcium and parathyroid hormone levels and larger adenomas. These patients might be given 1,25-dihydroxyvitamin D preoperatively to increase calcium absorption and shorten the time of symptomatic hypocalcemia.

▶ *This is a very interesting entity, and when you see it you will never forget it. Some years ago, I saw a young man with severe hyperparathyroidism who, after removal of a large adenoma, had intractable hypocalcemia for nearly 48 hours because of the "hungry bone" syndrome.*

The Epidemiology of Disseminated Nontuberculous Mycobacterial Infection in the Acquired Immunodeficiency Syndrome (AIDS)

Horsburgh CR Jr, Selik RM
Am Rev Respir Dis 139:4–7, January 1989 **1–34**

The AIDS epidemic is carrying with it an epidemic of disseminated nontuberculous mycobacterial infection, which occurs when an immunocompromised person is exposed to a ubiquitous infectious agent that is relatively nonvirulent for normal hosts. More than 2,000 infections were reported to the Centers for Disease Control in 1981–1987, and all but 4% were caused by the *Mycobacterium avium* complex. The patients were not more compromised immunologically than those with other opportunistic infections, but they survived a shorter time. As it is not practical to avoid exposure to these agents, efforts are needed to detect infection at an early stage and to treat it effectively.

▶ *Before the AIDS epidemic, there were only 78 published reports of disseminated nontuberculous mycobacterial infections. That's all changed now. Of the nontuberculous mycobacteria, the* avium *complex leads the list. As I'm sure you know, treatment is still less than optimal in this condition.*

Invasion of the Central Nervous System by *Treponema pallidum:* Implications for Diagnosis and Treatment

Lukehart SA, Hook TW III, Baker-Zander SA, et al
Ann Intern Med 109:855–862, Dec 1, 1988 **1–35**

Of 40 untreated patients with primary and secondary syphilis, nearly 1 in 3 had *Treponema pallidum* isolated from the cerebrospinal fluid (CSF). Also, 2 of 3 patients with early latent syphilis and 3 of 15 with late latent syphilis had VDRL-reactive spinal fluid. Although concurrent HIV infection did not relate to the presence of *T. pallidum,* all 3 patients with secondary syphilis from whom the organism was isolated and who failed to respond to treatment were HIV-seropositive at the time or seroconverted during follow-up. At a minimum, all syphilitic patients should be tested for HIV infection, and the CSF should be examined in those who are HIV-positive.

▶ *As you may recall, in 1989 we pointed out that the natural history of neurosyphilis was being altered by concurrent HIV infection (*Roundsmanship '89, *pp 36–37). This paper follows up on this theme and demonstrates that central nervous system invasion by* T. pallidum *is very common in early syphilis, even independent of HIV infection. The authors also raise the point that the current therapeutic recommendations for penicillin may be ineffective in patients with early syphilis who also have HIV infection.*

Endocrine Complications of the Acquired Immunodeficiency Syndrome

Aron DC
Arch Intern Med 149:330–333, February 1989 **1–36**

Even though endocrine dysfunction has not been a striking clinical feature of AIDS, all of the endocrine glands may be affected, whether by infectious agents, neoplasms, or the drugs used to treat infections. The most serious abnormalities (Table

TABLE 4.
Major Endocrine Complications in AIDS

Gland	Complication	Most Likely Causes
Adrenal	Cortisol and aldosterone deficiency	Opportunistic infection or ketoconazole
Pituitary	Syndrome of inappropriate antidiuretic hormone	Pulmonary or central nervous system infection or drugs
Thyroid	Euthyroid sick	Systemic illness
Pancreatic islets	Hypoglycemia	Pentamidine, inanition, or sepsis
Testis	Hypogonadism	Hypothalamic deficiency secondary to systemic illness or ketoconazole
	Gynecomastia	Ketoconazole
Parathyroid	Hypocalcemia	Systemic illness or hypomagnesemia

(Courtesy of Aron DC: *Arch Intern Med* 149:330–333, February 1989.)

4) are adrenocortical insufficiency caused by cytomegalovirus infection or ketoconazole therapy; hypoglycemia consequent to pentamidine therapy; and hyponatremia of diverse origin. Although the pancreas is often involved by infection or neoplasm, hyperglycemia is not a frequent sequel.

▶ *Last year, in 1989 (*Roundsmanship '89, *pp 37–38), we pointed out the association of adrenal insufficiency and AIDS. This interesting article follows up on this association and points out a number of other endocrine abnormalities found in patients with AIDS. As can be seen in Table 4, abnormalities occur in virtually every endocrine organ.*

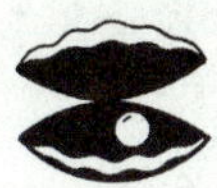

In the bedside evaluation of coma the key to differentiation of structural from metabolic causes is in the eye examination. The pupillary light reflexes are preserved with metabolic coma and lost with most structural causes. Dysconjugate eye movements suggest a structural cause.

Intestinal Infections in Patients With the Acquired Immunodeficiency Syndrome (AIDS): Etiology and Response to Therapy

Smith PD, Lane HC, Gill VJ, et al
Ann Intern Med 108:328–333, March 1988 **1–37**

A specific pathologic cause of diarrhea was found in 17 of 20 homosexual males with AIDS. Compared with 10 patients lacking diarrhea, they had lost more weight, had fewer helper-induced lymphocytes, and had more extraintestinal opportunistic infections. Only 1 non-diarrheic patient had an enteric pathogen. The long list of pathogens included cytomegalovirus, *Entamoeba histolytica*, *Cryptosporidium*, *Salmonella*, and *Giardia lamblia*. Ten of the 16 patients given antimicrobial therapy improved symptomatically. When an AIDS patient has diarrhea, it will not do to accept the "idiopathic" designation without a thorough work-up.

▶ *Various diarrhea syndromes are extremely common in patients with AIDS. Etiologic agents are multiple. Although cryptosporidium is found in the AIDS patients, you can see there are a huge number of other important organisms that also can be pathogenic. This article summarizes the results in 20 patients and outlines the appropriate therapy for each type of infectious diarrhea.*

Survival Experience Among Patients With AIDS Receiving Zidovudine: Follow-Up of Patients in a Compassionate Plea Program

Creagh-Kirk T, Doi P, Andrews E, et al
JAMA 260:3009–3015, Nov 25, 1988 **1–38**

Zidovudine, formerly known as azidothymidine, was made available to nearly 5,000 AIDS patients who had *Pneumocystis carinii* pneumonia. Survival after 44 weeks was 73% and approached 90% in patients who were in relatively good condition at the time treatment began. Adverse effects included serious anemia and granulocytopenia, each in about 10% of patients. Because those who are not yet severely ill stand to gain the most from zidovudine therapy, the drug should be given at even earlier stages.

▶ *This study further evaluates the use of zidovudine (AZT) in patients with AIDS. In patients using this therapy, survival at 44 weeks was 88%. This is obviously a very sobering way of looking at the data. In fact, AIDS is a lethal disease, and all of the evidence points to the fact that AZT has only a modest effect on prognosis. The side effects are not trivial, and we are just hoping for better things ahead in the treatment of this disease.*

Thrombotic Thrombocytopenic Purpura in Patients With the Acquired Immunodeficiency Syndrome (AIDS)-Related Complex: A Report of Two Cases

Nair JMG, Bellevue R, Bertoni M, et al
Ann Intern Med 109:209–212, Aug 1, 1988 **1–39**

Two patients, an intravenous drug abuser and a homosexual, had both the classic picture of thrombotic thrombocytopenic purpura and evidence of AIDS-related complex. The latter patient had extensive angiofollicular proliferation in the bone marrow and lymph nodes (Fig 1–12). Both patients entered remission after exchange plasmapheresis and treatment with antiplatelet agents and high-dose steroids. This association

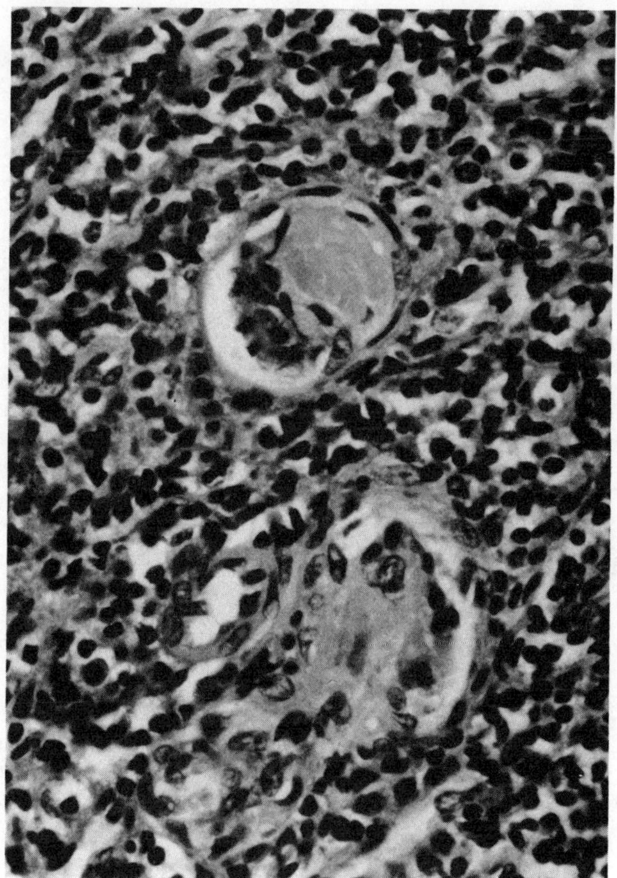

Fig 1–12
Lymph node with microthrombi within the capillaries. Hematoxylin and eosin; original magnification, ×250. (Courtesy of Nair JMG, Bellevue R, Bertoni M, et al: *Ann Intern Med* 109:209–212, Aug 1, 1988.)

is probably more than coincidental; AIDS and AIDS-related complex are well known to be related to other immune disorders.

▶ *Here is another clinical entity reported in connection with HIV. Interestingly, thrombocytopenia also has been associated with HIV positivity. Whether the latter association has to do with the frequency of intravenous drug administration, alcoholism, or other factors remains to be delineated. Who knows what disease we may report next year?*

Treatment of Infections Associated With Human Immunodeficiency Virus

Glatt AE, Chirgwin K, Landesman SH
N Engl J Med 318:1439–1448, June 2, 1988 **1–40**

Eventually, most AIDS patients contract *Pneumocystis carinii* pneumonia; in more than half of them it is the first opportunistic infection. Pentamidine isethionate or trimethoprim-sulfamethoxazole (TMP/SMX) is used initially, but newer approaches such as dapsone plus TMP are being tried. In addition, primary prophylaxis may prove worthwhile for high-risk patients. Toxoplasmosis in AIDS patients is treated with pyrimethamine and sulfadiazine. Amphotericin B is the mainstay for cryptococcal infection. Tuberculosis is treated as in other patients, but variants such as *Mycobacterium avium* and *Mycobacterium intracellulare* frequently caused disseminated disease and may be difficult to treat; experimental regimens hold some hope here. Many forms of herpesvirus infection can occur: mucocutaneous herpes simplex infection is treated with acyclovir orally; gastrointestinal disease and retinitis caused by cytomegalovirus infection may respond to ganciclovir, but pneumonia unfortunately does not.

▶ *The basic principles that the authors elucidate are worth repeating: (1) Fungal parasitic and viral infections as seen in AIDS patients are rarely curable. (2) Most HIV-associated infections result from endogenous reactivation and do not represent a threat to other persons. (3) Infections are rarely single. (4) The observed frequency of certain fungal or parasitic infections depends on the prevalence of asymptomatic infection in the local population. (5) Certain bacterial infections are seen only in HIV-associated diseases. (6) Infections associated with HIV disease are severe.*

Human Immunodeficiency Virus Infection in Hemophiliac Patients: A Three-Year Prospective Evaluation

Daul CB, deShazo RD, Andes WA
Am J Med 84:801–809, May 1988 **1–41**

Half of a series of heterosexual hemophiliacs were already seropositive for HIV when first assessed, and one third had per-

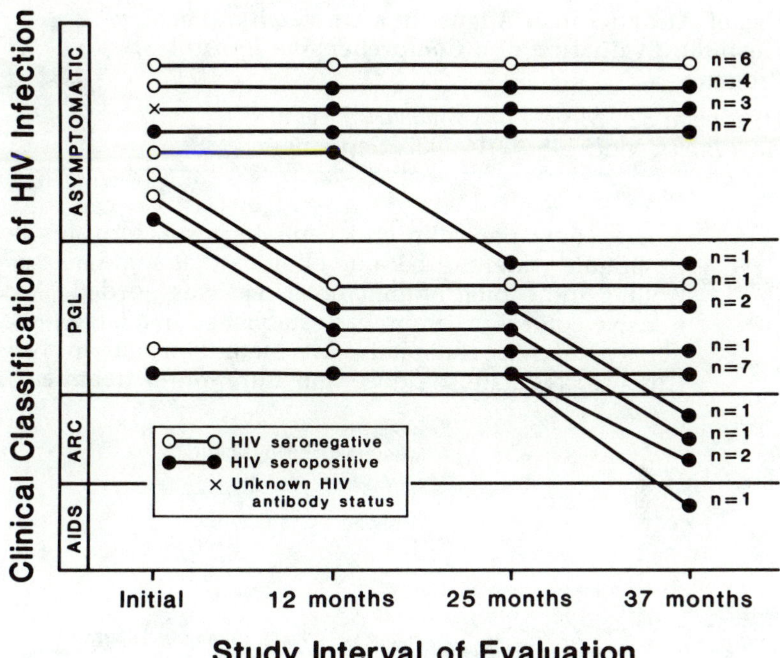

Fig 1–13
Clinical course and serologic evidence of HIV exposure of hemophilic patients. *Bars,* clinical history of each patient or group of patients; *n,* number of patients in each category. (Courtesy of Daul CB, deShazo RD, Andes WA, et al: *Am J Med* 84:801–809, May 1988.)

sistent generalized lymphadenopathy. Nine others seroconverted during follow-up, and 80% ultimately were seropositive (Fig 1–13). Lymphadenopathy developed in 6 patients during an average follow-up of 3 years. Four patients had progression to AIDS-related complex and AIDS developed in 1. Seropositive patients who remained asymptomatic had progressively abnormal lymphocyte function over time regardless of the number of CD4+ cells in the peripheral blood.

▶ *Hemophilia is a chronic disease that has become even more complex recently with its association with AIDS. A substantial number of patients have become HIV positive, or AIDS-related complex and even the full-blown disease have developed from the prolonged administration of factor concentrate therapy. The only good news is that seropositive individuals, compared with homosexuals, seem more likely to have the minor syndromes related to AIDS.*

Use of Antimicrobial Agents in a University Teaching Hospital: Evaluation of a Comprehensive Control Program

Hirschman SZ, Meyers BR, Bradbury K, et al
Arch Intern Med 148:2001–2007, September 1988 **1–42**

When new penicillin and cephalosporin derivates began to proliferate widely, it became obvious that some means of controlling in-hospital antimicrobial use was needed. A comprehensive control program was established in a large tertiary university teaching hospital—Mt Sinai Hospital in New York City—to regulate the dose and duration of treatment. An in-

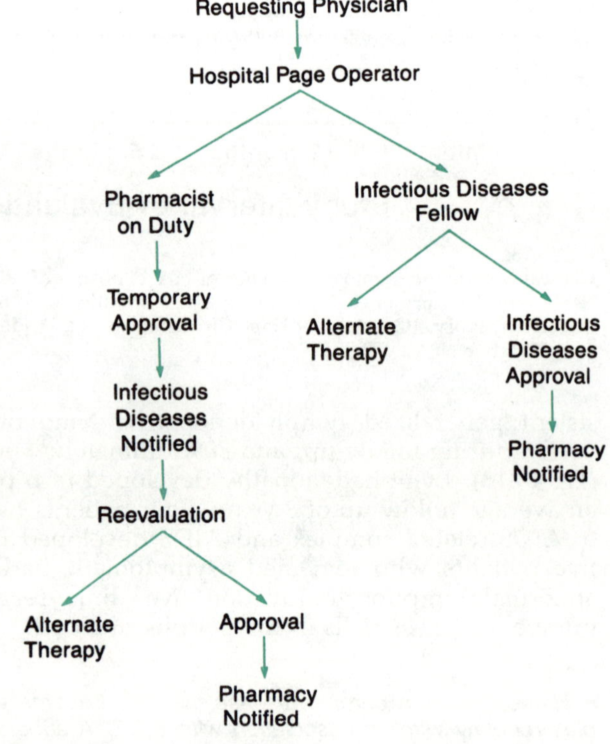

Fig 1–14
Outline of system for obtaining approval for use of restricted antimicrobial agents under present program. (Courtesy of Hirschman SZ, Meyers BR, Bradbury K, et al: *Arch Intern Med* 148:2001–2007, September 1988.)

fectious disease specialist had to approve the use of restricted drugs (Fig 1–14). Ongoing surveillance of drug use is an essential part of the program. Pharmacy costs for antibiotics fell by nearly a half million dollars in the first year of the program, and gross savings in the following year exceeded $200,000. In addition, there are ancillary savings such as less intravenous equipment and nursing time, and less pharmacist time for preparing drugs.

▶ *When one cost accounts hospital drug expenditures, antibiotics are clearly at the top of the list. This paper points out an excellent model that is not only efficacious from the fiscal standpoint but is medically sound. Obviously, certain ego-type problems are involved, but it is a plan worth considering. You certainly could reduce drug resistance this way. On the other hand, one might have to have Henry Kissinger as the administrator.*

Reading the Tuberculin Skin Test: Who, When, and How?

Howard TP, Solomon DA
Arch Intern Med 148:2457–2459, November 1988 **1–43**

Eight hundred healthy individuals had the standard Mantoux test with 5 tuberculin units of PPD injected intradermally in the volar forearm. The presence of any induration after 24 hours was 83% sensitive and 88% specific for traditional readings. Just over a third of the persons with induration read their own tests as positive, and the predictive value of a self-interpreted negative reading was only 78%. The PPD test should be read by a trained person, and decisions on individual patients must be based on readings at 48–72 hours.

▶ *I love to throw in some simple straightforward clinical maneuvers such as reading the tuberculin test. Howard and Soloman do a very nice job of evaluating more than 800 volunteers who were tested. They confirmed that one must evaluate the skin test at 48–72 hours, and that 24 hours is not good enough. Further, a patient's own measurements aren't worth anything.*

Prospective Study of Infections in Indwelling Central Venous Catheters Using Quantitative Blood Cultures

Benezra D, Kiehn TE, Gold JWM, et al
Am J Med 85:495–498, October 1988 **1–44**

More than a quarter of 500 central venous catheter placements were attended by catheter-related infection, and there were 88 episodes of catheter-related sepsis. Sixty percent of 54 septic episodes were controlled by antibiotic therapy. Tunnel infections were less readily controlled than exit site infections, and often it proved necessary to remove the catheter. *Pseudomonas* was responsible for many of these resistant infections, so that if this organism is present the catheter should be removed. Otherwise, antibiotics and local care may well suffice.

▶ *It seems that everyone is using an indwelling central venous catheter, and it is important to have evaluated the natural history of infectious complications associated with this foreign body. The main thing to remember is that catheter-related infections caused by* Pseudomonas *or polymicrobic organisms have a poor prognosis. One should be constantly thinking about these iatrogenic complications.*

Cytomegalovirus Pneumonia After Bone Marrow Transplantation Successfully Treated With the Combination of Ganciclovir and High-Dose Intravenous Immune Globulin

Emanuel D, Cunningham I, Jules-Elysee K, et al
Ann Intern Med 109:777–782, Nov 15, 1988 **1–45**

Ten patients with leukemia or congenital immune deficiency who contracted cytomegalovirus (CMV) pneumonia after allogeneic bone marrow transplantation received the antiviral drug ganciclovir combined with high-dose intravenous immune globulin. All 10 responded, and 7 were alive and well 6–13 months after treatment. In marked contrast, none of 11 patients given ganciclovir or immune globulin alone survived. The combination has substantially altered the outcome of CMV pneumonia in these patients.

▶ *The antiviral agent, ganciclovir, has been used in the treatment of CMV pneumonia. This particular study combined the antiviral agent with high-dose intravenous immune globulin, with encouraging results.*

Remember that CMV occurs in AIDS patients and in a number of other settings in which the patient is immunocompromised.

Acyclovir Treatment of the Chronic Fatigue Syndrome: Lack of Efficacy in a Placebo-Controlled Trial

Straus SE, Dale JK, Tobi M, et al
N Engl J Med 319:1692–1698, Dec 29, 1988 **1–46**

Chronic fatigue syndrome, with diffuse pain, tender lymph nodes, difficulty in concentrating, and depression, has been a therapeutic mystery. Because some data have suggested a role for Epstein-Barr virus (EBV), acyclovir was tried in 27 adults who had debilitating fatigue for 7 years on average. Three patients became nephrotoxic and were withdrawn from the trial. The others did not improve more often when given acyclovir than when given placebo, and the outcome did not relate to changes in EBV antibody titer or circulating immune complexes.

▶ *As noted, the chronic fatigue syndrome is characterized by debilitating fatigue, diffuse pains, sore throat, tender lymph nodes, decreased ability to concentrate, and, at times, depression. The existence of this syndrome has been debated for a long time; currently, it seems inescapable that it really does exist. In this study the authors gave acyclovir because of a previous suggestion of a relationship of this disease to EBV infection. Unfortunately, it had no effect. Although preliminary impressions suggested that the drug provided temporary benefit in this syndrome, this placebo-controlled study did not bear this out.*

Cryptococcal Infection of the Nervous System

Yu YL, Lau YN, Woo E, et al
Q J Med 66:87–96, January 1988 **1–47**

Eleven of 18 patients seen in 10 years with cryptococcal infection of the central nervous system had 1 of several active illnesses predisposing them to infection, but not AIDS. Two thirds of patients complained of fever, headache, and a stiff neck. Papilledema was seen in 8 patients, but only 3 had seizures. The India ink cerebrospinal fluid preparation demonstrated cryptococci in all but 3 patients. Despite intravenous treatment with amphotericin B and 5-fluorocytosine orally, 7 patients died. Three others relapsed but responded to a further course of treatment.

▶ *Cryptococcosis is, like so many infectious diseases, increasing in prevalence because of AIDS. Yet the disease does occur in seemingly nonimmunocompromised individuals as well. The diagnosis is usually made with India ink preparation and examination of the spinal fluid and treatment is with amphotericin B and 5-fluorocytosine. The prognosis is worse in immunocompromised patients.*

Enterococcal Bacteremia: Clinical Features, the Risk of Endocarditis, and Management

Maki DG, Agger WA
Medicine 67:248–269, July 1988 **1–48**

Enterococcal bacteremias are seen increasingly often. Other organisms were isolated along with enterococci in more than a third of 150 patients seen in a 14-year period. Serious underlying medical disease, usually malignancy, was the rule. Thirteen patients had endocarditis. The most common extracardiac sites of infection were an intra-abdominal or surgical wound, the urinary tract, a burn wound, and a vascular catheter. Nosocomial infections predominated in all of these groups, except that only 1 of 13 patients had nosocomial endocarditis. Nearly half of the patients died in the hospital, but those with endocarditis had a lower case-fatality rate. Appropriate antimicrobial treatment lowered mortality. It remains critically important to operate on local foci of infection and to remove an infected intravascular device.

▶ *The enterococci are the predominant aerobic streptococci of the bile and female genital tract and thus could be a common source of infection. This review indeed points out the various clinical manifestations of enterococcal bacteremia with special emphasis on bacterial endocarditis. This is not an easy organism to eradicate.*

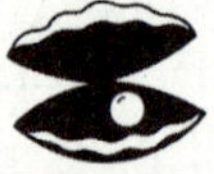

If osteomyelitis develops after a nail injury through a tennis shoe, it is likely to be caused by *Pseudomonas aeruginosa*.

Detection of Circulating Tumor Necrosis Factor After Endotoxin Administration

Michie HR, Manogue KR, Spriggs DR, et al
N Engl J Med 318:1481–1486, June 9, 1988 **1–49**

There may be a close association between induction of tumor necrosis factor and septicemia in animals, but the factor is inconsistently present in critically ill patients with gram-negative bacterial infections. When 21 normal individuals received endotoxin intravenously in a dose of 4 mg/kg, plasma levels of tumor necrosis factor increased by about sevenfold within 3 hours. Peak production correlated with flulike symptoms, an increase in white blood cells, and ACTH production. Pretreatment with ibuprofen lessened all of these responses but not the increase in circulating tumor necrosis factor. Neither interleukin-1 nor gamma interferon changed after endotoxin infusion. Ibuprofen and related drugs probably act indirectly by decreasing cytokine-mediated stimulation of the cyclooxygenase pathway. Treatments aimed at preventing cytokine production or end-organ responses may succeed only if used early when cytokines start to form.

▶ *In the past decade a number of new and important cytokines have been identified. Most intriguing of all may be the so-called tumor necrosis factor (cachectin), a 17-kd polypeptide. This substance, which may be responsible for a number of findings seen with gram-negative sepsis, is under intense investigation.*

Oesophageal Ischaemia in Motility Disorders Associated With Chest Pain

MacKenzie J, Belch J, Land D, et al
Lancet 2:592–595, Sept 10, 1988 **1–50**

What actually causes chest pain in patients who have diffuse esophageal spasm or a "nutcracker" esophagus? It is probably not esophageal muscle spasm, which often does not coincide with pain. When 9 patients and 21 normal persons were challenged by infusing water at 7 C through the lower esophagus, rewarming took significantly longer in the patients. Ischemia is a probable cause. As even the normal blood supply of the esophagus is sparse, any compromise could lead to both pain and dysmotility.

▶ *Recently, a lot of good work has been done in assessing esophageal motility. In this study from Glasgow the authors evaluate the mechanism of the severe pain seen with either esophageal spasm or the "nutcracker" esophagus. The data indicated that the pain is, in fact, of ischemic origin. The mechanism of this ischemia remains to be delineated but obviously has clinical implications for agents such as calcium channel blockers and related compounds.*

Campylobacter pylori Antibodies in Humans

Perez-Perez GI, Dworkin BM, Chodos JE, et al
Ann Intern Med 109:11–17, July 1, 1988 **1–51**

Campylobacter pylori is a gram-negative bacterium of the upper gastrointestinal tract that may be a useful marker of gastritis. Application of an enzyme-linked immunosorbent assay (ELISA) to nearly 400 patients and control sera showed that gastritis was associated with higher mean IgA and IgG titers. A positive result in both assays was more than 90% sensitive and specific for histologic gastritis. Antibody was rare in normal persons younger than age 20 but was found in more than half of those aged 60 or more. *Campylobacter pylori* antibody was not specifically associated with bacterial enteritis, acute pancreatitis, or inflammatory bowel disease. Whether it is a direct cause of gastritis or peptic ulcer remains an open question.

▶ *The plot thickens. Last year we discussed the possible association of* C. pylori *infections and the ulcer diathesis. This year we have an elegant ELISA that demonstrates the presence of antibodies against* C. pylori *in a substantial number of patients with acute gastritis. This is becoming a more fascinating issue every day.*

The Effects of Alcoholism on Skeletal and Cardiac Muscle

Urbano-Marquez A, Estruch R, Navarro-Lopez F, et al
N Engl J Med 320:409–415, Feb 16, 1989 **1–52**

Just what happens to cardiac and skeletal muscle in alcoholics? More than 40% of 50 asymptomatic alcoholic men had impaired

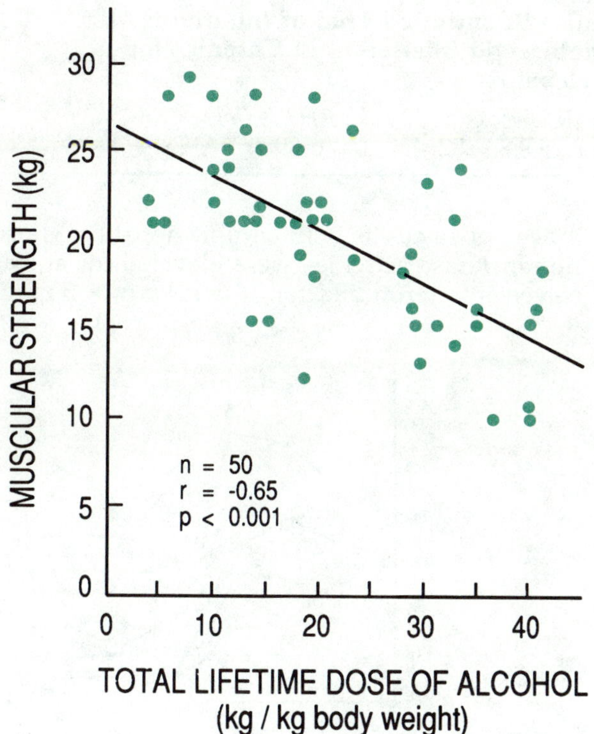

Fig 1–15
Correlation between the total lifetime consumption of ethanol and muscular strength in 50 alcoholic patients. (Courtesy of Urbano-Marquez A, Estruch R, Navarro-Lopez F, et al: *N Engl J Med* 320:409–415, Feb 16, 1989.)

deltoid muscle strength, and those who had consumed the most alcohol in their lives were the weakest (Fig 1–15). About half of the muscle biopsy specimens showed myopathic changes. The cardiac ejection fraction was lower than in healthy controls, and patients with cardiac dysfunction had changes of cardiomyopathy on endomyocardial biopsy. As was true of skeletal muscle, the lifetime dose of ethanol correlated inversely with ejection fraction. An important question is when a reversible lesion changes to necrosis with loss of muscle tissue.

▶ *For many years it has been known that chronic alcoholism can be associated with both skeletal muscle damage and a cardiomyopathy. This, the best recent study in this area, seems to make it clear that alcohol is toxic to skeletal muscle in a dose-dependent fashion. The next step is to define the molecular events that lead to skeletal muscle disorder.*

Randomized Controlled Trial of Interferon Alfa (Lymphoblastoid Interferon) in Chronic Non-A Non-B Hepatitis

Jacyna MR, Brooks MG, Loke RHT, et al
Br Med J 298:80–82, Jan 14, 1989 **1–53**

Seven of 14 adults with chronic hepatitis whose aspartate aminotransferase activities were elevated for at least 6 months received interferon alfa for 16 weeks in a final dose of 3 mega-

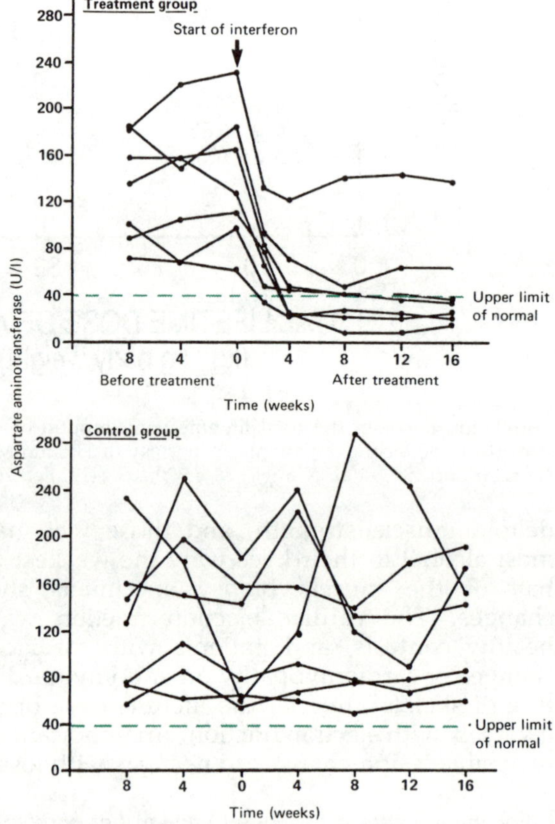

Fig 1–16
Serum aspartate aminotransferase activities (U/L) over time in treated and control patients with chronic non-A, non-B hepatitis. (Courtesy of Jacyna MR, Brooks MG, Loke RHT, et al: *Br Med J* 298:80–82, Jan 14, 1989.)

units 3 times a week. Serum enzyme levels fell rapidly to normal in treated patients but remained elevated in controls (Fig 1–16). Side effects were minor; all patients tolerated the treatment. Longer-term studies will show whether liver histology improves as well and whether improvement is lasting. Even if patients do relapse, ongoing low-dose treatment may be feasible.

▶ *These promising data give us hope for a therapy for patients with chronic non-A non-B hepatitis. As shown in Figure 1–17, there is a significant reduction in aspartate enzyme activity with the use of interferon alfa. It's also of interest that, as we go to press, announcements are being made that a vaccine for non-A non-B hepatitis is right around the corner.*

Colchicine in the Treatment of Cirrhosis of the Liver

Kershenobich D, Vargas F, Garcia-Tsao G, et al
N Engl J Med 318:1709–1713, June 30, 1988 **1–54**

Is colchicine, which inhibits collagen synthesis, helpful in treating cirrhosis of the liver? In a double-blind, placebo-controlled study of 100 patients, mostly with alcoholic or posthepatic cirrhosis, those treated actively received 1 mg of colchicine daily 5 days a week. Survival improved substantially (Fig 1–17); the median life expectancy tripled with colchicine therapy. More than half of the patients given active treatment remained alive after 10 years, compared with only 20% of controls. Also, 9 of 30 treated patients had histologic improvement and in 2 the liver appeared normal. Colchicine is a safe and effective treatment for patients with mild to moderate hepatic cirrhosis.

▶ *These investigators from the Nutritional Institute in Mexico City performed this study because of previous experience demonstrating that colchicine decreases fibrosis and hepatic functional abnormalities in rats with carbon tetrachloride-induced cirrhosis. The results are startling. We have not had available any type of therapy that is truly effective in preventing or attenuating hepatic disease in patients with cirrhosis. There was even histologic evidence of improvement, as well as the marked difference in survival. I am not sure what to say other than we probably need some confirmatory evidence, but it looks good at this point.*

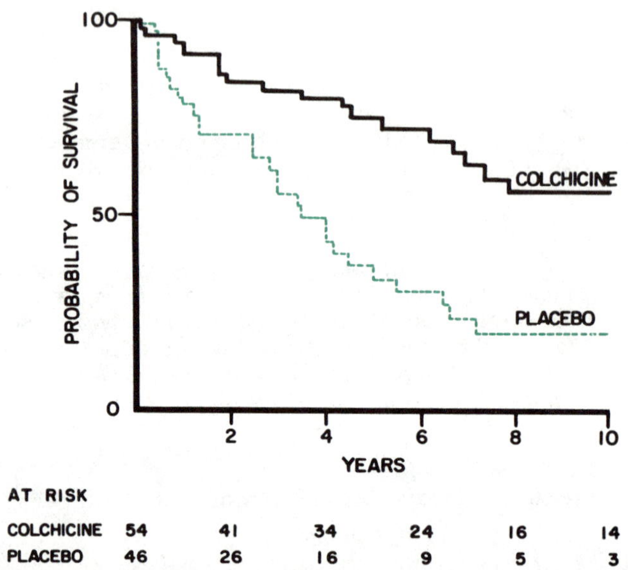

Fig 1–17
Survival curves based on reported deaths from any cause in the colchicine and placebo groups—a life-table depiction of the proportion of patients surviving in each treatment group. The curves end at 10 years because of the small number of patients at risk after this time; formal analysis of the efficacy of treatment included all deaths after 10 years until the end of the study. (Courtesy of Kershenobich D, Vargas F, Garcia-Tsao G, et al: *N Engl J Med* 318:1709–1713, June 30, 1988.)

Improvement of Hepatic Encephalopathy Treated With Flumazenil

Grimm G, Ferenci P, Katzenschlager R, et al
Lancet 2:1392–1394, Dec 17, 1988 **1–55**

Because increased GABAergic tone may be a factor in hepatic encephalopathy, the benzodiazepine antagonist flumazenil was evaluated in 17 patients with liver failure in whom conventional measures were ineffective. The stage of encephalopathy improved in 12 of 20 episodes when patients received varying doses of infused flumazenil, usually 15 mg in 3 hours. Most often, however, patients deteriorated within 4 hours after treatment. Several patients who failed to respond at all had clinically evident cerebral edema. The drug might prove more effective if given early in the course of encephalopathy.

▶ *Investigators continue to try to define the mechanism of altered mental status in patients with hepatic encephalopathy. Recent studies have shown that hepatic encephalopathy may be associated with an increase in the gamma aminobutyric acid inhibitory neurotransmitter system. In this context, the benzodiazepine antagonist flumazenil was given to 17 patients with hepatic encephalopathy. In most studies there was evidence of improvement in mental and somatosensory evoked potentials. This is encouraging, but we need many more studies before this becomes standard therapy.*

Fragmentation of Bile Duct Stones by Extracorporeal Shock Waves: A New Approach to Biliary Calculi After Failure of Routine Endoscopic Measures

Sauerbruch T, Stern M, and the Study Group for Shock-Wave Lithotripsy of Bile Duct Stones
Gastroenterology 96:146–152, January 1989 **1–56**

Eight percent of patients referred for endoscopic bile duct stone extraction were eligible for extracorporeal shock-wave lithotripsy (Table 5). Stones were cleared completely from the bile ducts in 86% of patients after a median of 4 days. Three fourths of the patients required only a single treatment. Most side effects were mild, but 2 patients died, 1 of an intra-abdominal hematoma that could have been caused by lithotripsy or other surgery. Two other patients required emergency surgery. Future studies will show whether comparable results can be achieved with energy levels not requiring anesthesia.

TABLE 5.

Criteria for Eligibility
Bile duct stones not amenable to routine endoscopic measures.
Sphincterotomy of the papilla of Vater performed.
No coagulation disorders.
Successful positioning trial of the calculi in the Dornier kidney lithotripter HM3.
No lung tissue, cysts, gas-filled bowel loops, vascular aneurysms, or calcified vessels in the shock-wave focal zone.

(Courtesy of Sauerbruch T, Stern M, and the Study Group for Shock-Wave Lithotripsy of Bile Duct Stones. *Gastroenterology* 96:146–152, January 1989.)

▶ *Here we have another use for the lithotripter. The results of this multicenter trial are encouraging. The main side effects include biliary and abdominal pain, gross hemobilia, hematoma of the skin, and in 1 instance each, gallbladder empyema and rupture of a juxtapapillary diverticulum.*

How to Image the Gallbladder in Suspected Cholecystitis

Marton KI, Doubilet P
Ann Intern Med 109:722–729, Nov 1, 1988 **1–57**

Real-time ultrasonography and cholescintigraphy are sensitive and specific enough to have replaced oral cholecystography in assessing the gallbladder. Ultrasonography is the best way of diagnosing chronic cholecystitis, using oral cholecystography as a back-up procedure. When acute cholecystitis is suspected but ultrasound study is not definitive, cholescintigraphy is most informative and may be done first if the focus is specifically on cystic duct obstruction. A wide range of secondary imaging procedures is available: intravenous cholangiography, computed tomography, magnetic resonance imaging, and endoscopic retrograde cholangiopancreatography.

▶ *Drs. Marton and Doubilet have done an excellent job in bringing us up to date on the way one studies patients with cholelithiasis. Real-time ultrasonography is the most reasonable first procedure in those patients suspected of having gallbladder disease. When uncertainty remains, cholescintigraphy can be used. One will find in the same issue a position paper by the American College of Physicians on this topic.*

A Multicenter Comparison of Lovastatin and Cholestyramine Therapy for Severe Primary Hypercholesterolemia

Lovastatin Study Group III
JAMA 280:359–366, July 15, 1988 **1–58**

How does lovastatin, which strongly inhibits hydroxy-methylglutaryl coenzyme A reductase, compare with cholestyramine resin in the treatment of severe primary hypercholesterolemia? About 250 patients given a lipid-lowering diet received 12 g of cholestyramine resin or 20 or 40 mg of lovastatin twice daily.

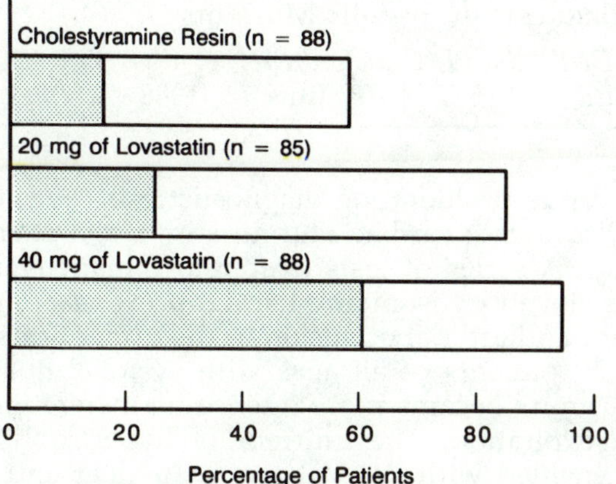

Fig 1–18
Percentages of patients with different degrees of response. *Shaded* and *open bars* indicate patients having at least a 20% reduction in low-density lipoprotein cholesterol levels at week 12; *shaded bar* only, those having at least a 40% reduction. Each drug was taken twice a day. (Courtesy of The Lovastatin Study Group III: *JAMA* 260:359–366, July 15, 1988.)

Lovastatin in the higher dose most effectively lowered levels of total cholesterol, low-density lipoprotein cholesterol (Fig 1–18), and apolipoprotein B. Only lovastatin reduced the very-low-density-lipoprotein cholesterol fraction and plasma triglycerides. Gastrointestinal effects were much less frequent with lovastatin therapy. Lovastatin combined with diet may lower coronary risk to an important degree in hypercholesterolemic patients.

▶ *This is an important study performed by individuals from at least 20 institutions. Lovastatin at a dose of 20 or 40 mg twice a day was associated with greater reductions in various lipid parameters than was cholestyramine. Further, the side effects were modest. Our experience with lovastatin is increasing, and the drug may one day be the first-line therapy for all patients with hypercholesterolemia. We will bring you up to date next year.*

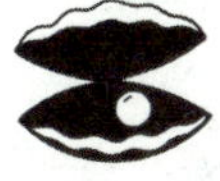

Smoking "crack" cocaine can cause acute diffuse alveolar hemorrhage with massive hemoptysis. This is usually mistaken for autoimmune-induced hemoptysis.

Bedside Diagnosis of Systolic Murmurs

Lembo NJ, Dell'Italia LJ, Crawford MH, et al
N Engl J Med 318:1572–1578, June 16, 1988 **1–59**

Despite proliferating diagnostic tests, bedside techniques can still evaluate cardiac murmurs in a cost-effective and accurate way. A series of tests (respiratory maneuvers, squatting, and leg elevation, isometric handgrip exercise, amyl nitrite inhalation, and arterial occlusion in the upper arms) were carried out in 50 patients of all ages with systolic murmurs. Right-sided murmurs became more intense on inspiration and less intense on expiration. The murmur of hypertrophic cardiomyopathy intensified with the Valsalva maneuver and when the patient moved from squatting to standing; it decreased with passive leg elevation and handgrip. The murmurs of mitral regurgitation and ventricular septal defect were augmented by handgrip and transient arterial occlusion, but decreased during amyl nitrite inhalation. Aortic stenosis was diagnosed by exclusion.

► *Here is an article for William Osler. This just goes to show that one can use a stethoscope and various maneuvers to diagnose the vast majority of murmurs. I just hope life never gets so sophisticated that an individual doesn't have to do a proper physical examination.*

Mental Stress and the Induction of Silent Myocardial Ischemia in Patients With Coronary Artery Disease

Rozanski A, Bairey CN, Krantz DS, et al
N Engl J Med 318:1005–1012, Apr 21, 1988 **1–60**

Stress responses to a variety of mental tasks were compared in 40 patients with coronary artery disease and 12 controls. In addition to mental arithmetic and a color-word task, the subjects told observers about their personal faults or undesirable habits, and they also read a passage on a neutral topic. Three fourths of patients had ventricular wall motion abnormalities while exercising and nearly as many during mental stress. Having to speak proved to be more stressful than thinking. Chest pain and ECG abnormalities occurred only when wall motion was compromised. What seems to be "spontaneous" myocardial ischemia may actually reflect uniquely stressful events of daily life, and this form of stress may be as important as exercise in triggering coronary events.

▶ *This article is both interesting and perplexing. The authors find that an emotionally arousing speaking task causes more frequent and greater regional wall motion abnormalities than less specific mental stress does. I wonder what that would mean to politicians or lecturers who don't feel comfortable during their speaking engagements. I wonder what it would mean to someone playing an agonizing game such as golf who had coronary artery disease. In any case, this paper shows unambiguous effects of mental stress on left ventricular function.*

Prevention of Coronary Artery Reocclusion and Reduction in Late Coronary Artery Stenosis After Thrombolytic Therapy in Patients With Acute Myocardial Infarction: A Randomized Study of Maintenance Infusion of Recombinant Human Tissue-Type Plasminogen Activator

Johns JA, Gold HK, Leinbach RC, et al
Circulation 78:546–556, September 1988 **1–61**

After opening up a coronary artery with intravenous recombinant tissue-type plasminogen activator (t-PA), will heparin maintain the patency, or is it better to continue t-PA infusion? In 52 patients who had a patent coronary artery after thrombolysis, 27 who were given heparin had reocclusion of the infarct-related artery, but none of those given maintenance t-PA did (and after 2 weeks they also had less residual stenosis). Clearly, t-PA infusion should be maintained after successful thrombolysis.

▶ *Once again, very gratifying results are reported with a thrombolytic agent. The $64 question, of course, is which streptokinase of these 2 (streptokinase or t-PA) is better. Certain data indicate that t-PA may be more effective (if it's used in the first 1–2 hours). Otherwise, at the moment we can't demonstrate any great differences between the 2 drugs. The other issue is that streptokinase is only 10% as expensive as t-PA. Using thrombolytic agents to manage acute myocardial infarction is an important area, and we'll certainly keep abreast of it in the next edition.*

Intravenous Streptokinase for Acute Myocardial Infarction: Effects on Global and Regional Systolic Function

Martin GV, Sheehan FH, Stadius M, et al
Circulation 78:258–266, August 1988 **1–62**

When 170 patients were randomized to receive intravenous streptokinase or standard treatment for myocardial infarction, after 10 days the vessel causing the infarct had opened in two thirds of the streptokinase group but in fewer than half of the controls. Myocardial wall motion was better in the infarcted region after thrombolysis, but the ejection fraction did not markedly improve. Even when thrombolysis does not directly save myocardium, reperfusion can improve function in remote areas and, as a result, global cardiac function will be better. This will especially help patients who have multivessel disease.

▶ *The cardiology group in Seattle has done an excellent study evaluating the use of streptokinase in patients with acute myocardial infarction. Intravenous streptokinase resulted in a higher patency rate and better left ventricular function even in areas remote from the site of infarction. Although the acute action of these thrombolytic agents is impressive, the long-term benefits and the effect on mortality are far from clear.*

Twelve-Year Follow-Up of Survival in the Randomized European Coronary Surgery Study

Varnauskas E, and the European Coronary Surgery Study Group
N Engl J Med 319:332–337, Aug 11, 1988 **1–63**

In the first 5 years of follow-up of 767 men with initially good left ventricular function, those assigned to surgery had significantly better survival. In the next 7 years the proportion of survivors declined more rapidly in the surgical group, but surgery remained the better therapy after 12 years (Fig 1–19). Despite the fact that 136 patients assigned to medical treatment underwent bypass surgery and 23 of those assigned to surgery did not. Surgery seemed to be somewhat more beneficial to older patients, those with markedly ischemic responses to exercise testing, and those with proximal LAD artery obstruction. The

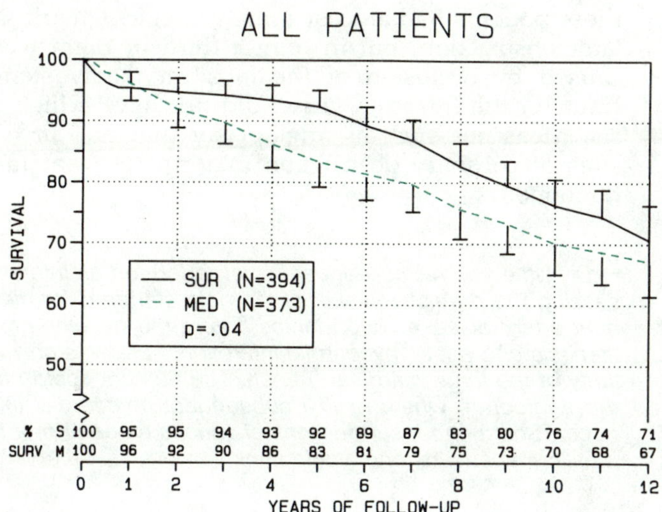

Fig 1–19
Twelve-year cumulative survival rates and 95% confidence intervals for all patients randomly assigned to either surgical treatment (SUR, S) or medical therapy (MED, M). *N*, number of patients; *% SURV*, percentage surviving. (Courtesy of Varnauskas E, and the European Coronary Surgery Study Group: *N Engl J Med* 319:332–337, Aug 11, 1988.)

findings to date do not favor an aggressive approach to patients at lower risk.

▶ *I know this topic gets confusing, but again I think that this is an excellent article. The fact is that survival is enhanced by surgery in patients who have multivessel disease, whereas in patients at lower risk it is not. This is clearly differentiated here.*

Can Coronary Angiography Predict the Site of a Subsequent Myocardial Infarction in Patients With Mild-to-Moderate Coronary Artery Disease?

Little WC, Constantinescu M, Applegate RJ, et al
Circulation 78:1157–1166, November 1988 **1–64**

Only if angiography can accurately predict the site of subsequent coronary occlusion will treatment aimed at sites of obstruction effectively prevent heart attacks. Twenty-nine of 42 patients who were examined before and within a month after acute infarction had a newly occluded coronary vessel. All of these patients had at least some vessel irregularity at the site of later obstruction, but in only a third of them was the infarct caused by occlusion of the most markedly stenosed artery. Usually, the infarcted vessel did not have a high-grade stenosis. Measures such as angioplasty that are directed solely at sites of coronary obstruction may not prevent many later infarctions.

▶ *Dr. Little and his colleagues have performed an interesting study assessing the predictive value of the gold standard for diagnosing coronary artery disease. Two months before the development of complete stenosis and acute myocardial infarction there was only a small irregularity of the large marginal branch. The authors could not predict from the angiogram where or if a subsequent myocardial infarction would occur. So much for suggestions of various types of prophylactic angioplastic maneuvers, one would think.*

A Prospective Randomized Trial of Outpatient Versus Inpatient Cardiac Catheterization

Block PC, Ockene I, Goldberg RJ, et al
N Engl J Med 319:1251–1255, Nov 10, 1988 **1–65**

Half a million cardiac catheterizations, including coronary angiography, are done each year in the United States. Would a less costly outpatient examination be safe? When groups of nearly 200 low-risk patients were compared, complication rates did not differ significantly. No patient in either group had a stroke or died. Total hospital charges were nearly $900 less in the outpatient group. Outpatient catheterization is indeed feasible for selected, clinically stable patients. Apart from substantial money savings, patients avoid the stress, risks, and inconvenience of a hospital stay.

▶ *Pretty soon, coronary bypass surgery is going to be an outpatient procedure. Seriously, this interesting study from the group at Massachusetts General presents the economic and medical rationale for doing elective cardiac catheterization as an outpatient procedure. The authors are also wise in urging caution before this approach becomes universally accepted and applied. Nevertheless, the study shows how a commonly used procedure can be carried out in a way that would save a lot of money in the health care arena.*

Reduction in the Rate of Early Restenosis After Coronary Angioplasty by a Diet Supplemented With n-3 Fatty Acids

Dehmer GJ, Papma JJ, van den Berg EK, et al
N Engl J Med 319:733–740, Sept 22, 1988 **1–66**

Eighty men having about 100 coronary artery lesions dilated received conventional antiplatelet therapy afterward; in addition, some were given 3.2 g daily of eicosapentaenoic acid. Restenosis was more than twice as frequent in the controls after 3–4 months (Table 6), and the symptomatic response accorded with angiographic findings. There were no important bleeding problems in the supplemented patients. There's nothing fishy about these results; a large-scale controlled trial is warranted.

▶ *What kind of a unappetizing diet will researchers come up with next? This important study looks at diet supplemented with n-3 fatty acids. The fact is that, at least in the male population at high risk for restenosis, dietary supplementation with these compounds reduced the occurrence of early restenosis. These studies obviously suggest more questions such as how this may relate to other aspects of coronary disease. The topic is certainly worth pursuing.*

TABLE 6.
Angiographic Results

Result	Control Group (N = 53)	Treatment Group (N = 50)	P Value
Luminal narrowing (%)			
Before angioplasty	80±13.3	78±13.7	NS
After angioplasty	29±14.0	25±15.1	NS
	P<0.001	P<0.001	
Vessels with			
Initial stenosis ≥90%	23	24	NS
Residual stenosis >35%	38	28	NS
Intimal dissection present	25	26	NS
Duration of follow-up (mo)	14.4±3.6	12.2±3.9	NS
Restenosis rate (per lesion, %)	36	16	0.026
Restenosis rate (per patient, %)	46	19	0.007

Plus-minus values, mean ±SD; *NS,* not significant; *mo,* months.
(Courtesy of Dehmer GJ, Papma JJ, van den Berg EK, et al: *N Engl J Med* 319:733–740, Sept 22, 1988.)

The Effect of Diltiazem on Mortality and Reinfarction After Myocardial Infarction

Multicenter Diltiazem Postinfarction Trial Research Group
N Engl J Med 319:385–392, Aug 18, 1988 **1–67**

What can we expect when heart attack victims are given diltiazem for 2 years? This large (2,500 patients) series from nearly 40 centers in the United States and Canada yielded a seemingly paradoxical finding: Fewer cardiac deaths and nonfatal reinfarctions occurred in patients without pulmonary congestion when they were given diltiazem, but in those with pulmonary congestion diltiazem therapy correlated with an increase in cardiac events. The net effect was neutral. What may be concluded from this study is that diltiazem is not appropriate for all survivors of myocardial infarction.

► *This multicenter trial was done well, but it did not show any impact of diltiazem on mortality or cardiac events in a population of patients with previous myocardial infarction. On the other hand, it must be noted that this was because of counterbalancing effects. Diltiazem did reduce cardiac events in patients with a normal ejection fraction, but the drug increased events in the small number of patients with left ventricular dysfunction. This is a well-known side effect of several calcium channel blockers.*

Relative Efficacy of Vasodilator Therapy in Chronic Congestive Heart Failure: Implications of Randomized Trials

Mulrow CD, Mulrow JP, Linn WD, et al
JAMA 259:3422–3426, June 17, 1988 **1–68**

The results of 28 randomized placebo-controlled trials of the use of vasodilators in chronic congestive heart failure (a disease that affects 2 million Americans) were evaluated. The studies, all lasting for at least a month and all double-blinded, included about 2,000 patients, predominantly middle-aged men with heart failure caused by ischemic coronary artery disease. The studies showed that angiotensin-converting-enzyme (ACE) inhibitors, nitrates, and alpha-antagonists were associated with functional improvement. The only agents that lowered mortality as well were the ACE inhibitors. In general, the best results were in patients with less severe heart failure.

▶ *In this meta-analysis highly specific criteria were used (randomized, placebo-controlled trials with clinical end points and treatment durations of 4 weeks or more collected from an extensive literature). The results are encouraging and suggest that most vasodilators, except for hydralizine, are effective in patients with congestive heart failure. The ACE inhibitors both decrease mortality and improve functional status.*

Lifetime Risk for Patients With Mitral Valve Prolapse of Developing Severe Valve Regurgitation Requiring Surgery

Wilcken DEL, Hickey AJ
Circulation 78:10–14, July 1988 **1–69**

As many as 5% of adults may have primary mitral valve prolapse. Although serious complications are infrequent, progressive myxomatous changes in the valve can produce severe mitral regurgitation. This study looked at 50 patients in New South Wales, Australia (population, 5.5 million) who required surgery for mitral regurgitation. The risk of mitral regurgitation rose sharply after age 50; interestingly, 75% of the patients were men. The number of operations for this complication will increase as the population ages.

▶ *When I was a medical student, no one had even recognized that mitral valve prolapse existed. Now we know that it is an extraordinarily common problem occurring in 2% to 5% of the population. Generally speaking, it is benign but, as this article demonstrates, in certain patients prolapse progresses to severe valve regurgitation. Surprisingly, the development of mitral insufficiency is more common in males, and it's important to remember that you just don't see it before the age of 50.*

Sickle Cell Heart Disease: Two-Dimensional Echo and Doppler Ultrasonographic Findings in the Hearts of Adult Patients With Sickle Cell Anemia

Simmons BE, Santhanam V, Castaner A, et al
Arch Intern Med 148:1526–1528, July 1988 **1–70**

Patients with sickle cell anemia live longer today, and complications such as cardiovascular disease are increasingly prominent in this group. Seven of 40 adults (mean age, 26) had mitral regurgitation, but in no case was it severe. Pulmonary hypertension was found in more than a third of the patients by echocardiography alone and in more than half on Doppler criteria. Only a fourth of patients had echocardiographic evidence of hypertrophied left ventricle. None of the findings related directly to the degree of anemia. As in other chronic anemias, left-sided volume overload leads to chamber enlargement, diastolic dysfunction, and increased pulmonary pressure.

▶ *One of the main points in the differential diagnosis of rheumatic fever (fever, cardiac murmurs, and arthralgia) is sickle cell anemia. This study from the cardiology group at Cook County Hospital points out once again the cardiovascular effects of sickle cell anemia. Interestingly, the study seems to indicate that the major effects result from the anemia per se rather than from anything specifically related to sickle cell disease. On the other hand, one does see at autopsy sludging in the pulmonary circulation and other abnormalities suggesting that pulmonary hypertension may occur as a major event in some patients.*

Open-Heart Surgery in Octogenarians

Edmunds LH Jr, Stephenson LW, Edie RN, et al
N Engl J Med 319:131–136, July 21, 1988 **1–71**

Soon 7.5 million Americans will be aged 80 and more, and perhaps 40% of these individuals have symptomatic cardiovascular disease. Aortic valve disease and coronary disease predominated in a series of 100 consecutive octogenarians and nonagenarians. There were 29 deaths within 3 months of surgery and 28 patients survived complications. About half of the patients lived for another 5 years (Fig 1–20). Cardiac symptoms resolved in the surviving patients, and those who died some time after operation were free of angina. Surgery does seem to be reasonable for elderly patients with advanced heart disease when alternatives have been exhausted. It is true, though, that mortality and complication rates are high.

▶ *At one time I would have never even considered the notion of reading an article entitled "Open-Heart Surgery in Octogenarians." Here it is, and the results are quite good. It is true, as the article suggests, that physiologic age and chronologic age are seldom synchronized and that physiologic age can't be quantified. Therefore, there are some patients, even those with substantial heart disease, who might be candi-*

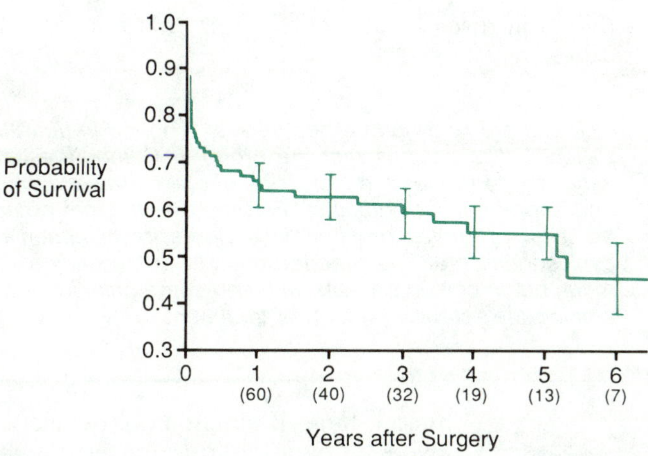

Fig 1–20
Actuarial survival curves for all patients. *Vertical bars* indicate standard errors of the estimate. Numbers of patients at risk are shown in parentheses. (Courtesy of Edmunds LH Jr, Stephenson LW, Edie RN, et al: *N Engl J Med* 319:131–136, July 21, 1988.)

dates for cardiac surgery when all else fails. In the series reported here, half of the patients had aortic valve disease and most of the others had isolated coronary artery disease. In any case, I think that these results from the University of Pennsylvania clearly indicate that in well-selected patients surgical procedures, even of a major type, can be efficacious in persons older than 80 years.

Heart-Lung Transplantation: Better Use of Resources

Hutter JA, Despins P, Higenbottam T, et al
Am J Med 85:4–11, July 1988 **1–72**

Acute rejection has not occurred in 31 patients given heart-lung transplants since 1984. Actuarial survival was 78% at 1 year and 70% at 2 years. Organized heart-lung transplantation depends on a method of procuring organs from distant sites. Adequate and simple techniques now are available for preserving the heart-lung allograft. Transbronchial lung biopsy makes it possible to accurately diagnose rejection at an early stage. Criteria for selecting recipients are widening, and cystic fibrosis patients now are potential recipients. It is hoped that more facilities will be established so that more patients with destructive lung disease can benefit from this now-established procedure.

▶ *These are some of the best results reported in heart-lung transplant patients. It is obvious that the group in Cambridgeshire has worked very hard to reduce the incidence of obliterative broncholitis, rejection, and superimposed infection. Further, the surgical procedure has become less complex, and immunosuppression has been improved in the cyclosporine era. The procedure is still in the early stage of development, but in certain patients with end-stage pulmonary disease it is becoming the established form of treatment.*

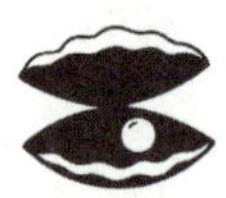

Buccal hyperpigmentation develops in patients given zidovudine prophylaxis. Because the frequency of Addison's disease is increased in AIDS patients, it is important to recognize that this classic physical sign of Addison's disease may be misleading.

The Pleura

Sahn SA

Am Rev Respir Dis 138:184–234, July 1988 **1–73**

This review of pleural disease is broad, deep, and incredibly comprehensive! After the author discusses how pleural fluid forms and outlines diagnostic measures—from the simple chest x-ray examination to open pleural biopsy—he presents an account of specific diseases producing transudative effusions, with congestive heart failure, cirrhosis, and nephrotic syndrome being prime examples. The lengthy differential diagnosis of exudative pleural effusion begins with infections, among which fungal and parasitic effusions and the atypical pneumonias figure prominently. Then there are the 3 forms of malignant effusion (carcinoma, lymphoma, malignant mesothelioma); the many immunologic causes such as sarcoidosis and rheumatoid pleurisy; other inflammatory causes (pancreatitis, uremic effusion); and lymphatic disorders. The review concludes with iatrogenic pleural disease that, apart from the many drugs implicated, includes radiotherapy and esophageal sclerotherapy.

▸ *This superb article reviews virtually everything one might want to know about the pleura, the diseases that affect it, and diagnostic procedures used to differentiate the various causes of exudative and transudative pleural effusion. Even a nephrologist enjoyed reading this beautiful paper. You should read this in its entirety.*

Bronchiectasis: Update of an Orphan Disease
Barker AF, Bardana EJ Jr
Am Rev Respir Dis 137:969–978, April 1988 **1–74**

In bronchiectasis the subsegmental airways are permanently dilated, tortuous, and often partly obstructed by exudate. The peripheral airways are inflamed and can be filled with secretions. The focal form, often affecting a single segment or lobe, may be cured by resection. On the other hand, diffuse bronchiectasis usually is related to widespread pneumonia, as can result from aspiration; hypersensitivity; immune deficiency states; or genetic disorders such as cystic fibrosis. Bronchography is used mostly in focal disease, but it may allow a firm diagnosis in a patient with persistent bleeding if bronchoscopy is negative. It may also serve to guide chest physiotherapy to the most seriously affected regions.

▸ *As the article indicates, the predisposing etiologic factors are multiple and may vary from a necrotizing pneumonic process to dyskinesia of the tracheal bronchial cilia. Bronchography is still the gold standard to use in diagnosing this disease. One needs to remember that there are specific causes of bronchiectasis that are treatable, e.g., allergic bronchopulmonary aspergillosis.*

The Use of Theophylline in "Irreversible" Chronic Obstructive Pulmonary Disease: An Update
Hill NS
Arch Intern Med 148:2579–2584, December 1988 **1–75**

Theophylline has variable effects on gas exchange in patients with irreversible chronic obstructive pulmonary disease. It remains to be seen whether mucociliary transport improves. Part of the confusion arises over lack of an apparent relationship between objective and subjective responses to theophylline. It is true that several well-designed studies suggest symptomatic benefit even if objective improvement is lacking. This would seem to warrant a cautious trial of sustained-release anhydrous theophylline in these patients. As always with theophylline, close attention to possible drug interactions is essential.

▶ *The therapy used in patients with chronic obstructive pulmonary disease (COPD) is usually of little value. Further, the number of well-controlled trials in these complex patients are few and far between. This paper evaluates the literature on the topic of the theophylline therapy in patients with severe COPD. The results seem to indicate that there are some patients who indeed benefit from this therapy, and that a cautious therapeutic trial is warranted if one takes into account the individual factors that can affect drug metabolism. Whether this effect on selected patients results from an increase in respiratory drive, enhanced mucociliary clearance, improved cardiovascular function, or enhanced diaphragmatic contractility alteratons is not clear.*

Complications of Acute Respiratory Failure

Pingleton SK
Am Rev Respir Dis 137:1463–1493, June 1988 **1–76**

Basically, 2 types of patients are seen in acute respiratory failure (ARF): older patients with primary obstructive lung disease or restrictive dysfunction, and younger, previously healthy patients with secondary lung injury (adult respiratory distress syndrome). This comprehensive review begins with the pulmonary complications of ARF—embolism, fibrosis, and barotrauma—and the many problems that can arise from ventilation and monitoring. Three body systems often are affected adversely by ARF: the gastrointestinal tract (pneumoperitoneum, bleeding); the cardiovascular system (hemodynamic changes, arrhythmias); and the kidneys (acute renal failure, edema, hyponatremia). Also, there are infectious events, most prominently nosocomial pneumonia, and nutritional complications such as malnutrition and increased CO_2 production. As if these weren't enough, hematologic and endocrine complications and psychiatric problems may attend ARF.

▶ *Today, critical care medicine is more and more popular among graduating students, and this review helps to point out some of the complexities of this area. For all of the technology that you may see in an intensive care unit, never forget that any intervention brings with it all types of possible complications. It isn't that glorious to have all of these tubes in and out of every orifice. The Swan-Ganz catheter can cause air embolism, arrhythmia, pneumothorax, and pulmonary artery rupture, not to mention various infectious complications.*

Pulmonary Embolism in Outpatients With Pleuritic Chest Pain

Hull RD, Raskob GE, Carter CJ, et al
Arch Intern Med 148:838–844, April 1988 **1–77**

In this series, about 20% of 173 patients seen in the emergency room with pleuritic chest pain proved to have pulmonary embolism. Predetermined clinical variables, although 85% sensitive in diagnosing embolism, were highly nonspecific. Perfusion lung scanning was 100% sensitive and 73% specific for pulmonary embolism. When pulmonary angiography was added to perfusion scanning, with or without ventilation imaging and impedance plethysmography, specificity improved to 97% and sensitivity remained extremely high. If ventilation imaging and plethysmography are combined with perfusion lung scanning, only 25% of patients will require angiography. The latter method does remain the definitive test for pulmonary embolism, however.

▶ *The group at McMasters in Hamilton, Ontario, continues to do excellent clinical epidemiologic studies on pulmonary embolism. In this particular paper, the authors emphasize that 20% of 173 consecutive patients seen in their emergency room with pleuritic chest pain had a pulmonary embolism. They assess the specificity and sensitivity of varying tests and remind us once again that angiography is the gold standard.*

Randomised Controlled Trial of Recombinant Tissue Plasminogen Activator Versus Urokinase in the Treatment of Acute Pulmonary Embolism

Goldhaber SZ, Kessler CM, Heit J, et al
Lancet 2:293–298, Aug 6, 1988 **1–78**

A randomized trial compared recombinant tissue-type plasminogen activator (rt-PA) with urokinase in an attempt to replicate the good results achieved in an open study of about 50 patients with acute pulmonary embolism. A 100-mg dose of rt-PA, infused in 2 hours, was compared with a 24-hour urokinase protocol. After 45 patients the study ended: Not only was rt-PA demonstrably more effective, based on the 2-hour pulmonary angiogram, but complications were less frequent than with urokinase. Lung scan reperfusion at 24 hours improved comparably in the 2 groups. This rt-PA regimen could become the standard for thrombolytic treatment of acute pulmonary embolism.

► *Well, it's nice to have a study in which investigators use rt-PA for something other than myocardial infarction. In this study, the authors compared the recombinant product with urokinase, another thrombolytic agent. Although rt-PA was safer and more rapid in action than urokinase, it's far from clear whether rt-PA should be used in preference to heparin except in very severe situations. It also should be cautioned that the end point of this study was radiologic rather than clinical improvement.*

Lung Function and Exercise Performance in Hyperthyroidism Before and After Treatment

Kendrick AH, O'Reilly JF, Laszlo G
Q J Med 68:615–627, August 1988 **1–79**

Why are many hyperthyroid patients dyspneic? Methacholine challenge of 16 patients before treatment did not demonstrate significantly increased airway reactivity. Some patients had a lowered functional residual capacity and subnormal peak respiratory muscle pressures. The respiratory exchange ratio on exercise was abnormally high and the anaerobic threshold consistently subnormal. Exercise ventilation improved substantially after treatment, but the breathing pattern and anaerobic threshold were unchanged. Improvement probably reflected a lesser sensation of dyspnea.

► *Hyperthyroidism is truly a multisystem disease. This paper evaluates the mechanism of dyspnea in these patients. The respiratory muscles are weak and clearly improve after treatment. Further, although the dyspnea may improve rapidly, the various modalities of pulmonary function take longer to return to normal.*

Is Routine Urine Testing in Outpatient Clinics Useful?

Morgan AG
Br Med J 297:1173, Nov 5, 1988 **1–80**

Lest the mundane urinalysis be taken for granted in this era of high-tech medicine, a review of nearly 6,000 clinic patients found that 5% had positive urinalyses. In more than a third of the patients results were not expected from available information. In 30 of them, 0.5% of all those tested, new diagnoses were made from the dipstick findings. Eight of these patients were diabetic, 6 had prostatism and obstruction, and 3 had urinary infection. In other instances a newly discovered abnormality was not looked into further. Like any routine procedure, urinalysis is justified only if what it discloses is put to good use.

▶ *I love this paper. A nephrologist in Nottingham, England, carried out a prospective study of the ". . . rewards of routine analysis of urine." In an era when it's fashionable to say that screening tests are a waste of time, this seems to me to be of some value. As you note, 30 diagnoses were made because of the routine dipstick analysis of the urine. Included in this were 8 patients with diabetes mellitus. I won't begin to calculate any of the cost-benefit ratios and other such things. I just want to remind every medical student that the urinalysis is important.*

Red-Cell-Volume Distribution Curves in Diagnosis of Glomerular and Non-Glomerular Haematuria

Shichiri M, Hosoda K, Nishio Y, et al
Lancet 1:903–911, Apr 23, 1988 **1–81**

How does one decide, in the absence of obvious renal or systemic disease, whether hematuria is of gomerular origin? Distortion of glomerular red cells may provide an answer. Size distribution curves were obtained with an automated blood cell analyzer in urine samples from 150 patients with definite causes of hematuria. Normally, the red cell peak was at a larger volume than that of peripheral red cells, but in patients with glomerulonephritis it was nearly always at a much smaller volume. The usual "nonglomerular" distribution was found in all but 1 of 47 patients with lower urinary tract lesions other than infection. Patients with infection had either a "glomerular" or a mixed distribution; they excreted distorted and dysmorphic red cells. This rapid and reproducible assay may avoid the need for biopsy in some patients with hematuria.

▶ *Fairley and Birch published a paper (*Kidney Int *21:105–108, 1982) pointing out that red blood cells of glomerular origin were distorted, pyknotic, and had irregular shapes, as one might expect for cells going through a hypertonic milieu such as the renal medulla. I had concerns, however, about the sensitivity and specificity of using these concepts to differentiate glomerular from nonglomerular bleeding. This paper provides a quantitative method for delineating the difference between the glomerular and nonglomerular distribution of red cells, and I think it is a substantial addition to the literature.*

Aluminum Chelation Therapy in Dialysis Patients: Evidence for Inhibition of Haemoglobin Synthesis by Low Levels of Aluminium

Altmann P, Plowman D, Marsh F, et al
Lancet 1:1012–1015, May 7, 1988 **1–82**

Both a functional deficiency of erythropoietin and uremic toxins contribute to the anemia of end-stage renal disease. Can aluminum further depress hemoglobin synthesis in this setting? When 15 patients exposed to a low level of aluminum received the chelating drug deferoxamine for 3 months, *serum* aluminum levels tripled and the hemoglobin increased (Fig 1–21), along with mean cell volume and the mean cell hemoglobin concentration. It seems that even a modest accumulation of aluminum can markedly inhibit hemoglobin synthesis. There were no major complications from chelation therapy.

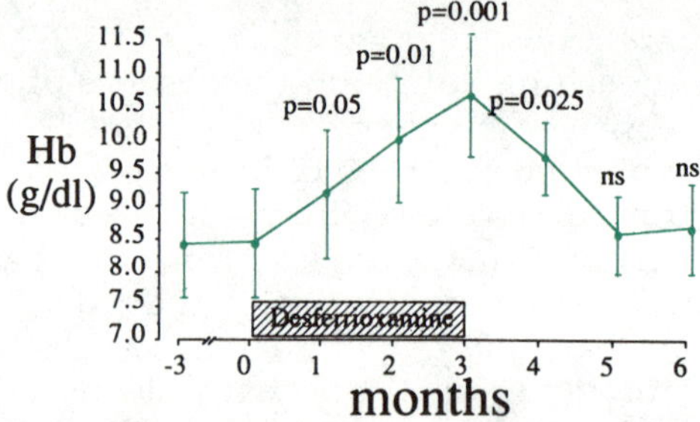

Fig 1–21
Effect of deferoxamine on hemoglobin concentration. *P* values refer to differences from baseline hemoglobin concentration. (Courtesy of Altmann P, Plowman D, Marsh F, et al: *Lancet* 1:1012–1015, May 7, 1988.)

▶ *The anemia of chronic renal failure has been studied extensively. In the hands of most individuals it has been found that a deficiency of erythropoietin is usually responsible. In this study a further problem, aluminum accumulation, seemingly plays a role. The data shown in Figure 1–22 indicate a clear relationship between infusion of deferoxamine and a rise in the serum hemoglobin concentration.*

Recombinant Human Erythropoietin Treatment in Pre-Dialysis Patients: A Double-Blind Placebo-Controlled Trial

Lim VS, DeGowin RL, Zavala D, et al
Ann Intern Med 110:108–114, Jan 15, 1989 **1–83**

This well-controlled study in 14 predialysis patients—adults with renal insufficiency and a mean hematocrit of 21%—

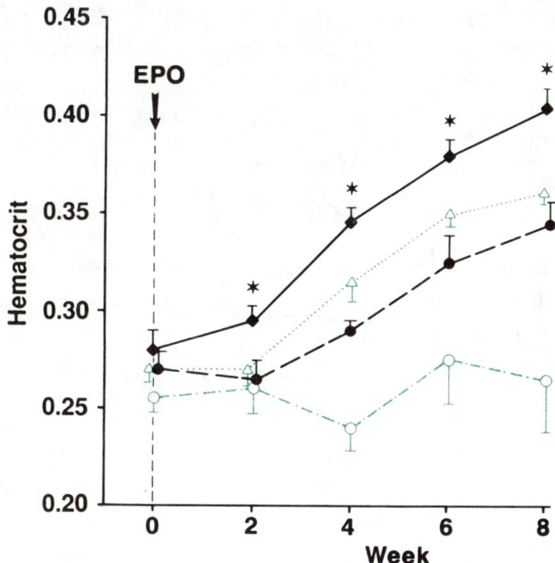

Fig 1–22
Effect of recombinant human erythropoietin (r-HuEPO) on the anemia of renal insufficiency. Three of 14 patients received placebo *(open circles)*, 3 received r-HuEPO, 50 U/kg *(filled circles)*, 4 received r-HuEPO, 100 U/kg *(triangles)*, and 4 received r-HuEPO, 150 U/kg *(diamonds)*. *Stars*, $P<.05$ to $P<.0001$ by ANOVA. There were significant differences between all groups except between the 50-unit and 100-unit groups. (Courtesy of Lim VS, DeGowin RL, Zavala D, et al: *Ann Intern Med* 110:108–114, Jan 15, 1989.)

showed that treatment with recombinant human erythropoietin for 8 weeks safely increases the hematocrit and red cell mass (Fig 1–22). Importantly, exercise tolerance improved and patients felt much better. No adverse effects were noted. The dose of erythropoietin was 50, 100, or 150 IU/kg, given intravenously 3 times a week.

► *As was reported in the 1989 edition (pp 12–13), recombinant human erythropoietin is efficacious in patients with chronic renal failure. The present study carries this a step further and points out the efficacy and safety of this recombinant product in predialysis patients. The drug is very expensive, however, and it is hoped that the Health Care Financing Administration will begin paying the costs for patients in chronic dialysis programs.*

Acute Rhabdomyolysis Associated With Cocaine Intoxication

Roth D, Alarcón FJ, Fernandez JA, et al
N Engl J Med 319:673–677, Sept 15, 1988 **1–84**

Among the myriad deleterious effects of cocaine abuse is rhabdomyolysis. A third of 40 such patients seen in 8 years (Fig 1–23) had acute renal failure, and 6 of them died. These pa-

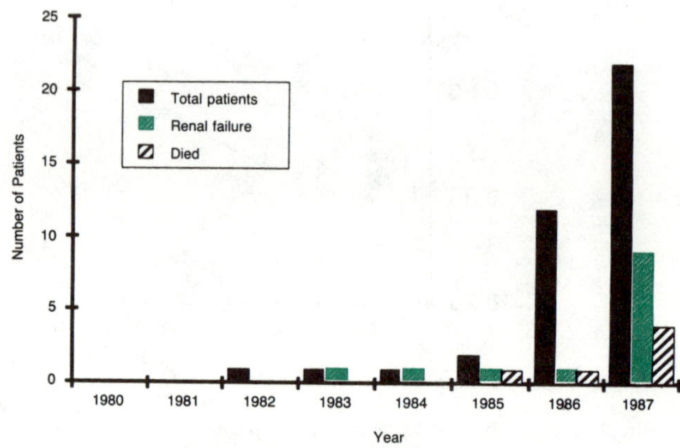

Fig 1–23
Patients hospitalized for cocaine intoxication with acute rhabdomyolysis, from 1980 through 1987, including those with renal failure and those who died. (Courtesy of Roth D, Alarcón FJ, Fernandez JA, et al: *N Engl J Med* 319:673–677, Sept 15, 1988.)

tients were inclined to be profoundly hypotensive and febrile at the outset, with a markedly elevated level of serum creatine kinase. All of the patients who died had disseminated intravascular coagulation. In addition, several patients in renal failure had marked liver dysfunction. All of those without renal failure survived.

▶ *In the 1989 edition we noted that one of the medical complications of cocaine abuse is sudden death. This article points out the marked increment in acute rhabdomyolysis and acute renal failure in cocaine addicts in the Miami area. Although many of these patients were taking other agents that also can cause rhabdomyolysis, the relationship between cocaine and rhabdomyolysis now seems to be quite clear.*

Contrast Nephrotoxicity: A Randomized Controlled Trial of a Nonionic and an Ionic Radiographic Contrast Agent

Schwab SJ, Hlatky MA, Pieper KS, et al
N Engl J Med 320:149–153, Jan 19, 1989 **1–85**

Does the experimental evidence that nonionic contrast agents are less nephrotoxic than ionic agents translate into clinical practice? When iopamidol and diatrizoate were compared in 443 patients requiring cardiac catheterization, serum creatinine

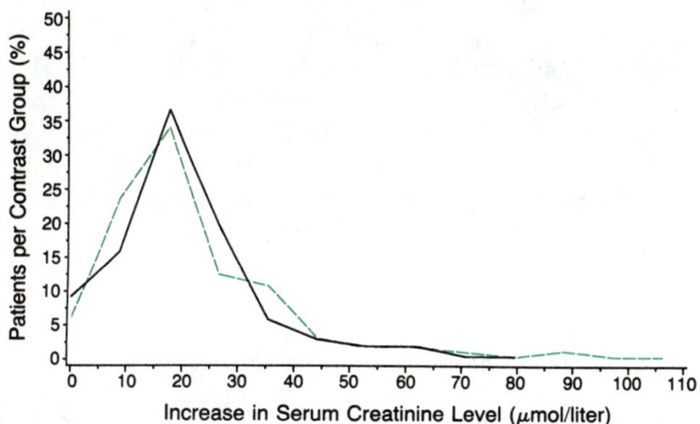

Fig 1–24
Peak increases in serum creatinine levels after administration of contrast agents. The percentage of patients is plotted against the maximal increase in creatinine level from baseline values. *Solid line,* 208 patients receiving iopamidol; *dashed line,* 235 patients receiving diatrizoate. (Courtesy of Schwab SJ, Hlatky MA, Pieper KS, et al: *N Engl J Med* 320:149–153, Jan 19, 1989.)

elevations were comparable with the 2 agents (Fig 1–24). Similar numbers of high-risk patients had a rise in the creatinine level of 44 μmol/L or more with the ionic and nonionic contrast materials. Especially considering the cost of nonionic agents, there generally is no advantage to using such agents to prevent renal injury.

▶ *The newly developed nonionic contrast materials are very expensive and gave promise of a diminished number of side effects, most notably renal function impairment. However, as shown by Figure 1–25, that is not the case.*

Endothelin: An Important Factor in Acute Renal Failure?

Firth JD, Ratcliffe PJ, Raine AEG
Lancet 2:1179–1181, Nov 19, 1988 **1–86**

Endothelin is a potent vasoconstrictor peptide that causes intense, long-lasting renal vasoconstriction in very low concentrations. Because hemodynamic changes probably are critical in early acute tubular necrosis, it is worth asking whether endothelin compromises renal perfusion in this setting. Angiotensin II has little effect on the glomerular filtration rate (GFR) in the isolated rat kidney, but a rise in endothelin from 100 to 800 pmol/L lowers the GFR by 90%. If, as seems likely, endothelin normally circulates in low concentration, hypotension and hypoxia could stimulate its release. A suggestive experimental finding: Pretreatment with a calcium entry blocker prevents ischemic acute renal failure. Endothelin apparently activates transmembrane calcium flux into vascular tissue.

▶ *Endothelin, the newest and hottest vasoactive peptide, is the most potent vasoconstrictor yet characterized. Recent work has suggested that it may be on a molar basis 5 times more potent than angiotensin II. This article evaluates that potency in light of the peptide's role in the pathogenesis of acute renal failure. The results are interesting but not conclusive. The pathogenesis of acute renal failure must be multifactorial. It will be interesting to follow the progress of the specific role of endothelin in this important clinical entity.*

Hemodynamic and Coagulation Responses to 1-Desamino[8-D-Arginine] Vasopressin in Patients With Congenital Nephrogenic Diabetes Insipidus

Bichet DG, Razi M, Lonergan M, et al
N Engl J Med 318:881–887, Apr 7, 1988 **1–87**

In congenital nephrogenic diabetes insipitus, a rare X-linked disorder, V_1-receptor vascular smooth muscle responses are intact, but the renal tubules with their V_2 receptors are resistant to arginine vasopressin and to dDAVP, an antidiuretic V_2-specific agonist. Infusion of dDAVP into patients with central diabetes insipidus as well as normal persons lowered the mean arterial pressure and increased the pulse rate, renin activity, and release of coagulation factors. Such changes did not occur in 7 males with congenital nephrogenic diabetes insipidus, and obligate carriers of the gene had only minimal responses (Fig 1–25). Apparently, there are extrarenal vasopressin V_2-like receptors that may be defective in this disease, and this may provide a means of identifying obligate carriers of the gene.

▶ *Recent studies have indicated that there are at least 2 sets of receptors responsive to the action of arginine vasopressin: V_2 cyclic AMP, dependent receptors that account for the antidiuretic effect of the peptide, and V_1 receptors, which seemingly are responsible for the vasoconstrictor action of the agent. In the study by Bichet and associates, the results would seem to indicate that there are extrarenal V_2-like receptors that may be defective in patients with congenital nephrogenic diabetes insipidus. This may not be a universal finding, however, and we will keep you up to date.*

Improvement of Renal Function With Selective Thromboxane Antagonism in Lupus Nephritis

Pierucci A, Simonetti BM, Pecci G, et al
N Engl J Med 320:421–425, Feb 16, 1989 **1–88**

Because patients with lupus nephritis excrete increased amounts of thromboxane B_2 in the urine, the vasoconstrictive effect of thromboxane A_2 may alter renal hemodynamics in this setting. In accord with this possibility, infusion of a thromboxane receptor antagonist led to a significant rise in inulin and para-aminohippurate clearances in 10 patients (Fig 1–26). Sodium excretion also increased, but arterial pressure was un-

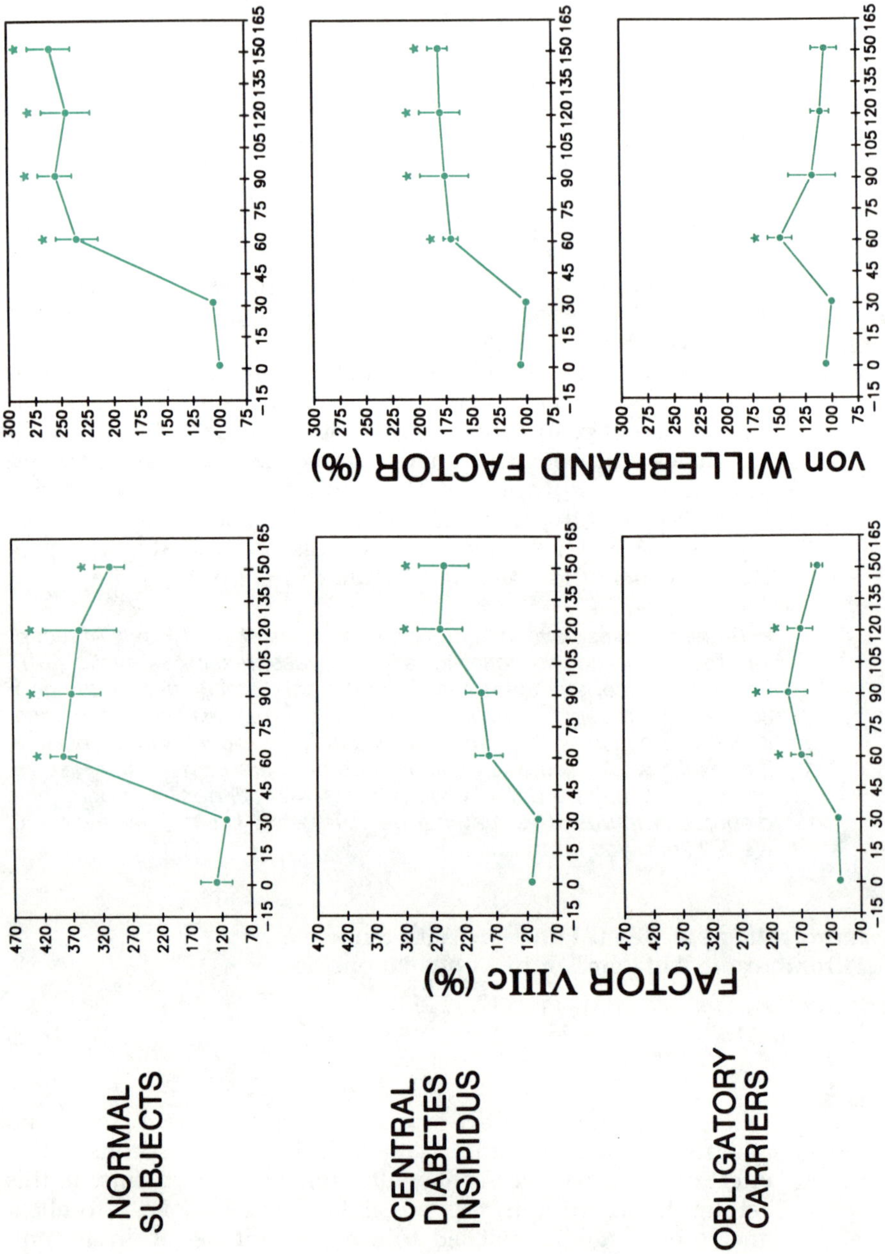

NORMAL SUBJECTS

CENTRAL DIABETES INSIPIDUS

OBLIGATORY CARRIERS

FACTOR VIIIc (%)

von WILLEBRAND FACTOR (%)

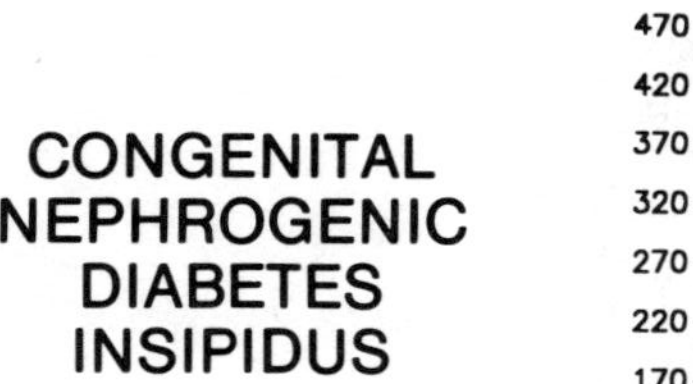

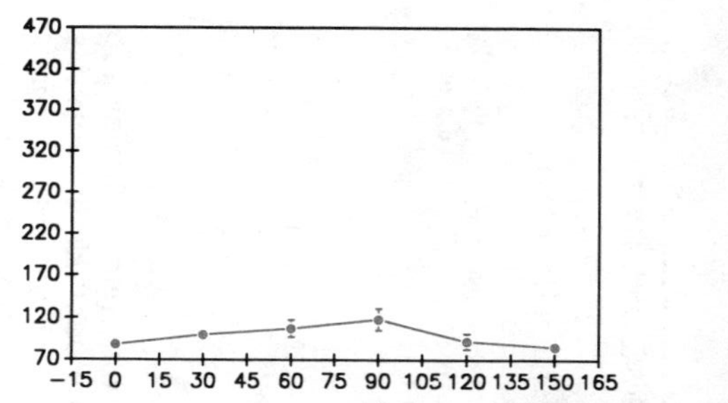

Fig 1–25
Factor VIIIc and von Willebrand factor responses to dDAVP infusion. All patients received the dDAVP infusion for 30–50 minutes. *Asterisks,* significant differences from baseline (values at 0 and 30 minutes). (Courtesy of Bichet DG, Razi M, Lonergan M, et al: *N Engl J Med* 318:881–887, Apr 7, 1988.)

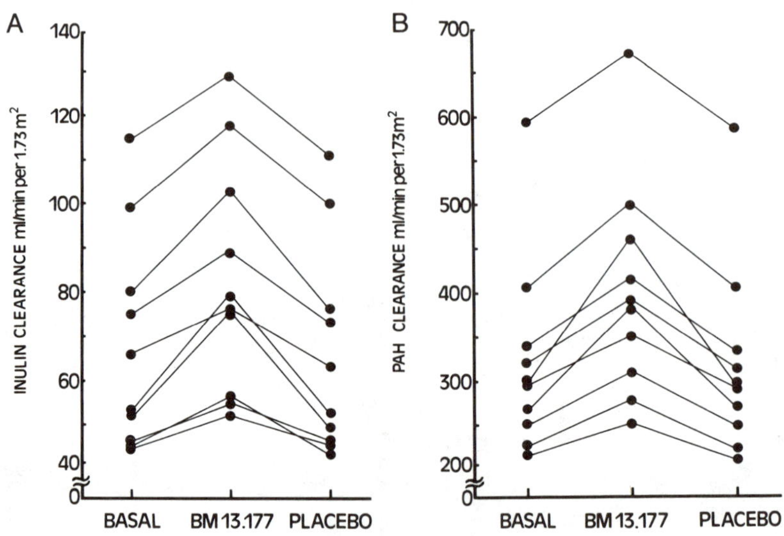

Fig 1–26
Individual inulin clearance rates **(A)** and para-aminohippurate (PAH) clearance rates **(B)** in 10 patients with lupus nephritis measured at baseline and during 48-hour continuous infusion of the thromboxane-receptor antagonist BM 13,177 or placebo. $P<.01$ for BM 13,177 vs. baseline and vs. placebo. (Courtesy of Pierucci A, Simonetti BM, Pecci G, et al: *N Engl J Med* 320:421–425, Feb 16, 1989.)

changed. The use of aspirin for 4 weeks did not alter either insulin clearance or the urinary thromboxane B_2 level. Safe and long-lasting receptor antagonists will be needed if these results are to find clinical application.

▶ *Recently, there have been a number of experimental studies suggesting that renal function impairment in lupus nephritis is caused, at least in part, by the potent vasoconstrictor thromboxane A_2. Figure 1–27 shows a clear increment in renal function when a specific inhibitor of thromboxane, BM 13,177, was given to a patient with lupus nephritis.*

Short Term Effect of Captopril on Microalbuminuria Induced by Exercise in Normotensive Diabetics

Romanelli G, Giustina A, Cimino A, et al
Br Med J 298:284–288, Feb 4, 1989 **1–89**

Nephropathy is an important cause of morbidity and mortality in diabetics. A study of the angiotensin-converting-enzyme inhibitor captopril in 54 patients with type I and type II diabetes showed a significant reduction in exercise-related albumin excretion compared with placebo. Blood pressure did not change significantly in these normotensive patients. Apparently, captopril can lower the renal intracapillary pressure, and it may thereby slow the progression of nephropathy when used early in the course of illness. It remains to be learned whether a reduction in microalbuminuria implies a lessening of structural glomerular disease.

▶ *This is confirmation of the important study discussed in the 1989 edition by Marre et al. (pp 14–15). The study shows that converting enzyme inhibition significantly reduced microalbuminuria induced by exercise in normotensive diabetics without affecting blood pressure. This once again raises the possibility that these agents may alter glomerular pressure independent of systemic pressure, a view that has obvious clinical implications for preventing the progression of renal disease.*

Natural Course of Penicillamine Nephropathy: A Long Term Study of 33 Patients

Hall CL, Jawad S, Harrison PR, et al
Br Med J 296:1083–1086, Apr 16, 1988 **1–90**

Penicillamine therapy is effective against active rheumatoid disease. It is therefore widely used, and its associated nephropathy continues to occur. In 33 rheumatoid patients in whom proteinuria developed during oral penicillamine therapy, proteinuria peaked a month after treatment ceased and resolved spontaneously within 18 months in nearly all patients. Creatinine clearance did not change appreciably (Fig 1–27, p 80). Most importantly, no patient required treatment for renal failure. The usual biopsy finding was membranous glomerulonephritis.

▶ *Penicillamine is now used fairly often in patients with complex and otherwise unresponsive rheumatoid arthritis. Thus renal damage has become a major problem. It has not been totally clear whether the renal dysfunction seen with penicillamine is reversible if the drug is discontinued. The present study seems to indicate clearly that this is the case, and it therefore makes a major therapeutic contribution to the literature.*

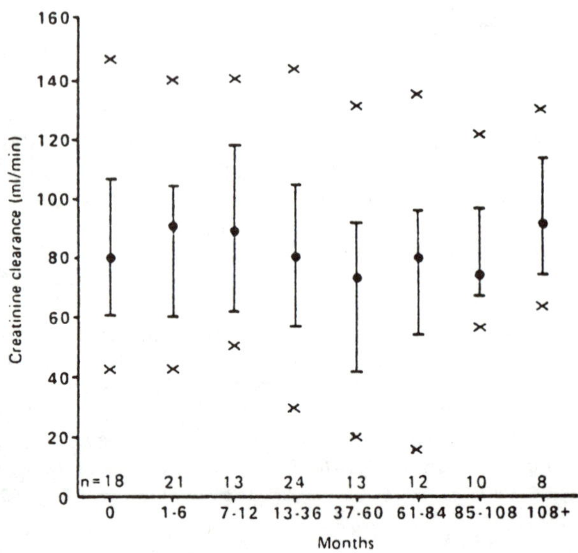

Fig 1–27
Creatinine clearance after penicillamine treatment stopped. Numbers of patients in parentheses. *Circles,* median; x, limit of range; *vertical bars,* interquartile range. (Courtesy of Hall CL, Jawad S, Harrison PR, et al: *Br Med J* 296:1083–1086, Apr 16, 1988.)

Microscopic Nephrocalcinosis in Cystic Fibrosis

Katz SM, Krueger LJ, Falkner B
N Engl J Med 319:263–266, Aug 4, 1988 **1–91**

Ion transport is abnormal in epithelial cells of the airways and sweat ducts in cystic fibrosis, so what about the kidney, an organ rather well adapted for ion transport? All but 3 of 38 autopsy renal specimens exhibited microscopic nephrocalcinosis, and this was present even in neonates. Calcium was seen within tubular mitochondria in the proximal convoluted tubules, but these cells generally were intact. Consistent with this finding, 5 of 14 cystic fibrosis patients were hypercalciuric. There may well be a primary abnormality of calcium metabolism in the kidneys in this disease.

▶ *I've always thought there ought to be some renal abnormality in cystic fibrosis. A number of investigators have studied chloride transport and other parameters of renal function, and it has been rare that any of them have found an alteration. Thus it is quite interesting that microscopic nephrocalcinosis was noted in these patients.*

Atheromatous Renal Disease

Meyrier A, Buchet P, Simon P, et al
Am J Med 85:139–146, August 1988 **1–92**

Thirty-two patients with renal failure associated with atheromatous kidney disease had been hypertensive for 10 years on average. Renal insufficiency was marked at presentation: The mean serum creatinine level was 6.8 mg/dL. Atheromatous renal artery stenosis was the chief factor in 22 patients. Ten had evidence of cholesterol embolism. Several patients were unsuitable for surgery for both anatomical and medical reasons. When feasible, reconstructive surgery was carried out and succeeded in 5 of 6 patients. The course of illness was related to the extent of atheromatous disease (Fig 1–28, p 82). This diagnosis is readily overlooked, but if it is made before irreversible renal atrophy and multivisceral compromise have developed, angioplasty or surgery is a possibility.

▸ *We tend to forget about atheromatous renal disease. It is common and easily overlooked. As described, it is not only caused by renal artery stenosis, but may also be associated with multiple stenosis of the intrarenal vasculature as well as cholesterol embolization. In our geriatric population it is becoming a bigger and bigger problem. Note Figure 1–29, showing progression of this entity.*

Echocardiographic Findings in Autosomal Dominant Polycystic Kidney Disease

Hossack KF, Leddy CL, Johnson AM, et al
N Engl J Med 319:907–912, Oct 6, 1988 **1–93**

Because cardiac murmurs are frequently noted in patients with autosomal dominant polycystic kidney disease, echocardiography, including Doppler analysis, was carried out in 163 patients as well as in 130 unaffected relatives and 100 controls. Mitral valve prolapse was found in fully 26% of the polycystic kidney group, 14% of the family members, and 2% of controls. Mitral and aortic regurgitation, as well as incompetence and prolapse of the tricuspid valve, also were more prevalent in patients with polycystic kidney disease (Fig 1–29, p 83). These findings support the concept of a systemic disease arising from disordered extracellular matrix formation.

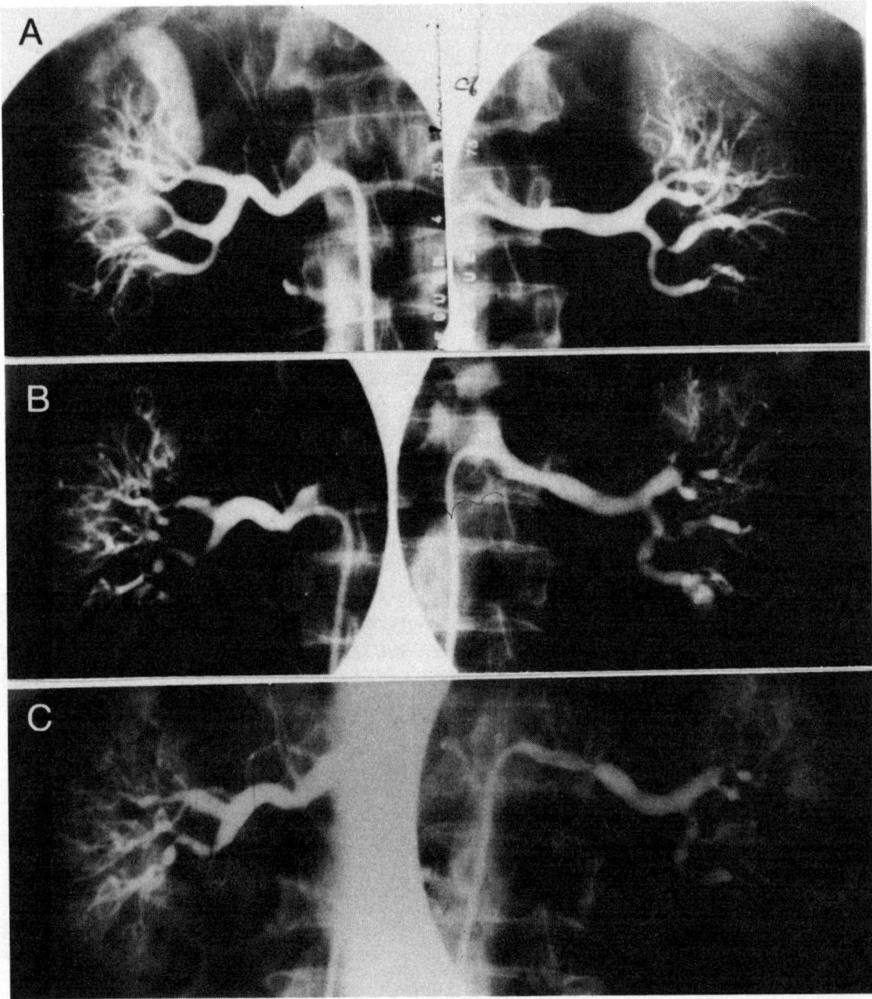

Fig 1–28
Development of atheromatous renal disease in a man, 43, with severe hypertension resistant to treatment with α-methyldopa, clonidine, and furosemide. **A,** early angiogram shows stenosis of the initial portion of the first division branches of the renal arteries. Malignant hypertension developed 2 years later with rapidly progressive renal insufficiency. Renal biopsy disclosed malignant nephrosclerosis. **B,** renal angiography revealed constitution of bilateral proximal stenoses of both main renal arteries. Maintenance hemodialysis was started. **C,** third angiogram obtained 1.5 years later shows distinct aggravation of all stenotic lesions. Some branches of the renal arteries are completely occluded with infarcts of the adjacent cortex. (Courtesy of Meyrier A, Buchet P, Simon P, et al: *Am J Med* 85:139–146, August 1988.)

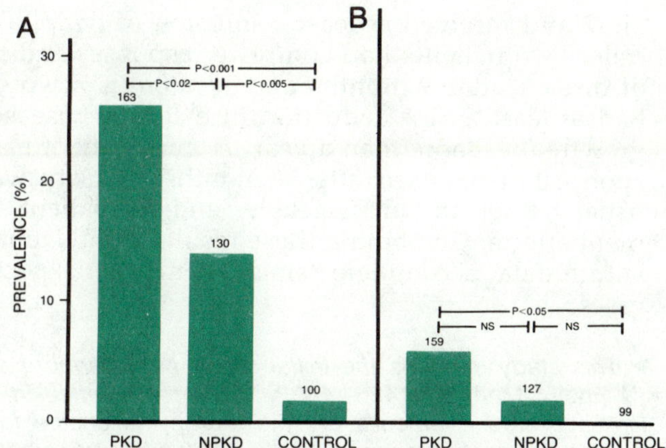

Fig 1–29
Prevalence of mitral valve prolapse **(A)** and tricuspidvalve prolapse **(B)** among patients with polycystic kidney disease (PKD), unaffected family members (NPKD), and controls. The *number* at the top of each column is the number of patients with satisfactory studies in each group. *P* values were determined by the chi-square test. (Courtesy of Hossack KF, Leddy CL, Johnson AM, et al: *N Engl J Med* 319:907–912, Oct 6, 1988.)

▶ *Lots of new information has been delineated recently concerning autosomal dominant polycystic kidney disease (ADPKD). This article clearly demonstrates the increased prevalence of mitral valve prolapse in patients with ADPKD. The finding suggests the systemic nature of the disease and supports the view that there is indeed a defect in the extracellular matrix in various tissue sites. The genetics of ADPKD is also under intense investigation. In another article in this issue of the* New England Journal of Medicine *(pp 913–918), Kimberling and associates delineate a second type of genetic abnormality in patients with this entity. Reeders in the* British Medical Journal *(292:851–853, 1986) initially demonstrated the close linkage of ADPKD to the alpha hemoglobin complex on the short arm of chromosome 16. Kimberling and his group found a totally different locus, indicating the heterogeneity of this disease.*

Metastatic Renal Cancer Treated With Interleukin-2 and Lymphokine-Activated Killer Cells: A Phase II Clinical Trial

Fisher RI, Coltman CA Jr, Doroshow JH, et al
Ann Intern Med 108:518–523, April 1988 **1–94**

Thirty-two patients with either metastatic renal cell cancer or unresectable disease were primed with recombinant interleukin-2 and received at least 1 infusion of lymphokine-activated cells. Two patients had complete responses and remained free of disease after 9 months and 12 months. Two other patients had at least a 50% reduction in extent of disease with no regrowth after more than a year. A third patient had a partial response but relapsed after 4 months. Toxicity was severe but usually brief and manageable, and no patient died of treatment effects. Combining these results with National Cancer Institute data, a complete remission may be expected in 10% of cases.

▶ *This study confirms the initial report of Rosenberg and colleagues (*N Engl J Med *313:1485–1492, 1985) that interleukin II and lymphokine-activated killer cells are the therapy of choice for patients with metastatic renal carcinoma. Our institution has been one of the centers involved in this study, and at least in some patients this approach is superior to any other known therapy. It must be recognized, however, that this therapy is extraordinarily expensive and results in a number of complications. Also, the most incredible capillary leak syndrome (peripheral edema and pulmonary edema) may develop. As a nephrologist, I have never come in contact clinically with anything quite like it.*

Regulation of Glomerular Filtration Rate in Chronic Congestive Heart Failure Patients

Cody RJ, Ljungman S, Covit AB, et al
Kidney Int 34:361–367, September 1988 **1–95**

The lowered renal blood flow in chronic congestive heart failure goes along with a reduced glomerular filtration rate (GFR) and impaired sodium and water excretion. In 34 such patients the GFR correlated directly with the cardiac index and also with renal blood flow (Fig 1–30). It correlated inversely with both systemic and renal vascular resistances. Older patients tended to have lower GFR and filtration fraction values. Renal blood flow alone accounted for two thirds of the observed variability in GFR. Renal function is fragile in elderly patients with chronic congestive failure.

▶ *It is well known that the GFR may fall dramatically in patients with severe congestive heart failure. This study further amplifies this phenomenon. Many studies have shown that the ratio of the GFR to renal plasma flow is increased in congestive heart failure because of preferential constriction of the efferent arteriole.*

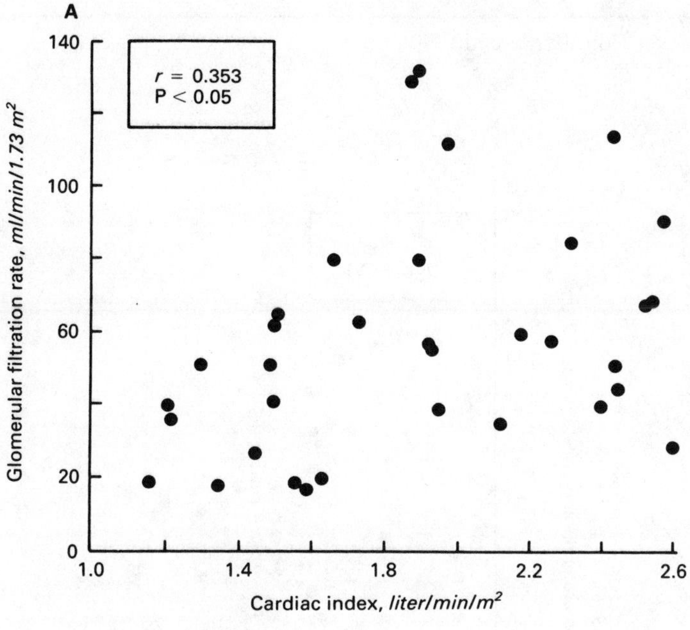

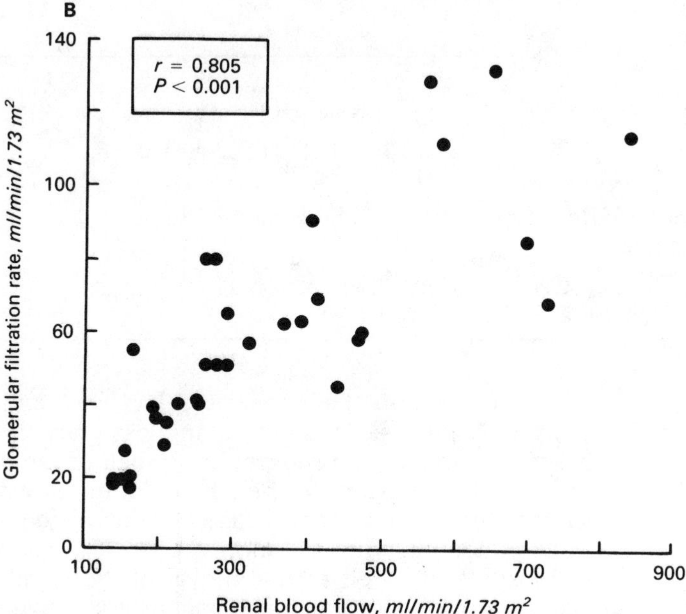

Fig 1–30
The hemodynamic correlates of the GFR in patients with congestive heart failure: cardiac index **(A)**, renal blood flow **(B)**, and renal fraction of cardiac output **(C)**. (Courtesy of Cody RJ, Ljungman S, Covit AB, et al: *Kidney Int* 34:361–367, September 1988.)

Continued.

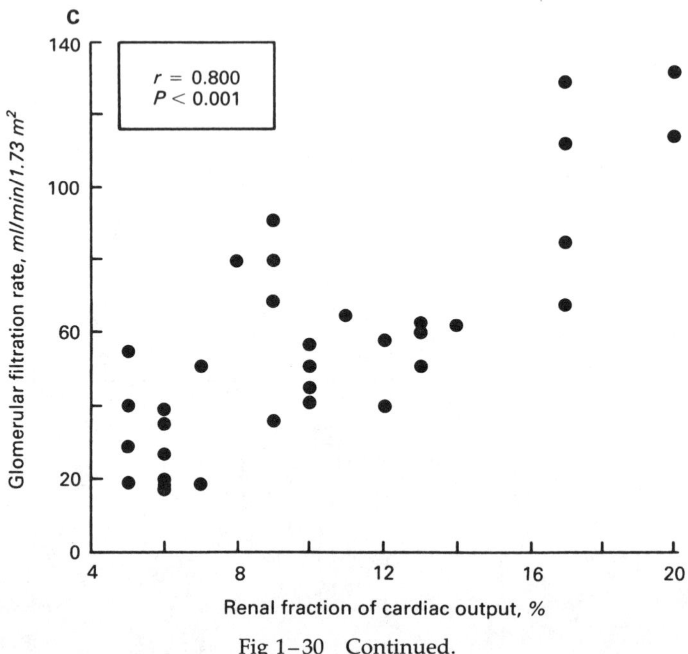

Fig 1–30 Continued.

Renovascular Hypertension: The Small Kidney Updated

Geyskes GG, Oei HY, Klinge J, et al
Q J Med 66:203–217, March 1988 **1–96**

Fifty-seven patients had renovascular hypertension with a small, poorly perfused kidney having less than 25% of total iodohippurate uptake on renography. In half of the patients with a totally occluded artery to the small kidney, attempted percutaneous angioplasty generally failed. It succeeded, however, in 22 of 28 patients having a stenotic vessel. Ten patients with bilateral lesions did well after removal of the small kidney and angioplasty of the contralateral renal artery. Salvage of a small kidney is important only when angioplasty of its artery is feasible. If the renal artery to the larger kidney is stenosed, it should be dilated. Residual hypertension usually responds to drug therapy.

► *Renal vascular hypertension is still a major problem to diagnose and treat. In the past decade, percutaneous transluminal angioplasty has become an important adjunctive therapy for this condition. This study seems further to confirm the usefulness of this modality of therapy in these complicated patients. Interestingly, it also further confirmed that cholesterol embolization is a common problem in elderly patients with atherosclerosis.*

The 1988 Report of the Joint National Committee on Detection, Evaluation, and Treatment of High Blood Pressure

1988 Joint National Committee
Arch Intern Med 148:1023–1038, May 1988 **1–97**

The latest version of the step-care approach to antihypertensive therapy (Fig 1–31) is more flexible than ever. It encourages more patient involvement, emphasizes quality of life, and addresses cost. Risk factor control is prominent and now encompasses the new cholesterol guidelines and use of calcium and fish oil supplements. After stepping up, one should step

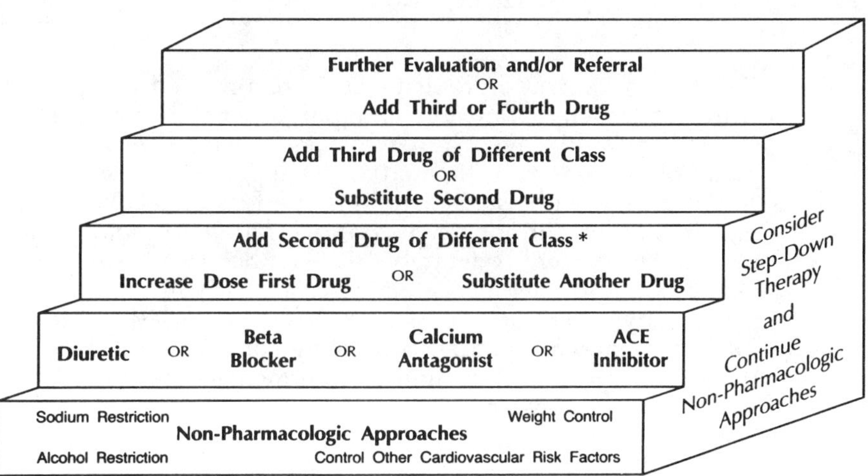

Fig 1–31
Individual step-care therapy for hypertension. For some patients, nonpharmacologic therapy should be tried first. If the blood pressure goal is not achieved, add pharmacologic therapy. Other patients may require pharmacologic therapy initially. In these instances, nonpharmacologic therapy may be a helpful adjunct. *ACE,* angiotensin-converting enzyme; *asterisk,* drugs such as diuretics, β-blockers, calcium antagonists, ACE inhibitors, α-blockers, centrally acting a_2-agonists, rauwolfia serpentina, and vasodilators. (Courtesy of 1988 Joint National Committee: *Arch Intern Med* 148:1023–1038, May 1988.)

down, if possible, with the aim of eventual drug withdrawal. The report discusses individualized approaches to antihypertensive management in many special situations, notably racial and ethnic minorities, pregnancies, the elderly, and patients having any of a long list of medical disorders.

▶ *Frequently, national committees do nothing but confuse things. I must say, however, that this report is a very good distillation of the complex treatment of hypertension. Although the step-care approach has seemingly been abandoned, Figure 1–32 certainly seems to bear some resemblance to a staircase. On the other hand, the new recommendations have created much more flexibility, and I think this is commendable.*

Raised Plasma Intact Parathyroid Hormone Concentrations in Young People With Mildly Raised Blood Pressure

Grobbee DE, Hackeng WHL, Birkenhäger JC, et al
Br Med J 296:814–816, March 19, 1988 **1–98**

Because hyperparathyroidism is more prevalent in persons with primary hypertension and parathyroid hormone is increased in middle-aged hypertensives, plasma levels of intact parathormone were estimated in 90 untreated persons aged 16–29 years with stable, mild hypertension. Levels were higher than in normotensive controls, but serum and urinary calcium levels were comparable. It may therefore be that circulating parathormone levels are increased early in the course of primary hypertension. Possible mechanisms include increased calcium in smooth muscle, promoting contractility and raising the peripheral resistance, and an intermediate effect on the renin-angiotensin system.

▶ *There have been a number of papers attempting to associate hyperactivity of the parathyroid gland with hypertension. In fact, it is fairly well known that hypercalcemia can be associated with accelerated hypertension. On the other hand, some studies suggest that an increased intake of milk is a protective factor in the development of hypertension. Be that as it may, this study, seemingly done in a careful manner, suggests that, as a group, hypertensive patients have a substantially higher basal level of parathyroid hormone.*

The Effects of Antihypertensive Agents on Serum Lipids and Lipoproteins

Lardinois CK, Neuman SL
Arch Intern Med 148:1280–1288, June 1988 **1–99**

If antihypertensive drugs adversely affect lipoproteins, this may counter the benefits of blood pressure reduction. Elevated triglycerides are reported in several studies of diuretic therapy. β-Blockers, especially nonselective agents, also can adversely affect lipid levels, and when combined with diuretics the effects are more pronounced. α-Adrenergic blockers, in contrast, favorably affect lipoprotein metabolism. If a thiazide diuretic fails to control blood pressure, a lipid-neutral agent should be added.

▶ *We are certainly in the era of reducing cholesterol at any cost. This article reviews the effects of various antihypertensive agents on lipid metabolism. It has been known for many years that diuretics modestly increase total cholesterol, at least in some clinical settings. This is because of increments in low-density and very-low-density lipoprotein. Also, certain β-adrenergic blocking agents decrease high-density lipoprotein. How one works around this is becoming more complex, and prospective studies are necessary to delineate whether these agents truly have a deleterious effect.*

2

Obstetrics and Gynecology

Maternal Weight Gain: Effect on Infant Birth Weight Among Overweight and Average-Weight Low-Income Women

Frentzen BH, Dimperios DL, Cruz AC
Am J Obstet Gynecol 159:1114–1117, November 1988 **2–1**

The effects on birth weight of maternal weight gain during pregnancy were compared in groups of 60–80 indigent women from the rural South who were 135% or more overweight or of average weight before pregnancy. Weight gain affected birth weight only in the average-weight group. Infant outcomes were similar in the 2 groups and, indeed, although birth weights differed in the expected direction, the difference was not significant. The degree of overweight is an important consideration, and recommendations for pregnancy weight gain should be tailored accordingly. It may be better to emphasize the quality of the diet than to suggest a minimum weight gain.

▸ *There have been several studies relating the infant's birth weight to the mother's weight gain during pregnancy. These have been of interest because we have seen a gradual increase in the number of macrosomic infants born to nondiabetic mothers. Part of this, I think, has been attributed to the significant increase in birth weight by the mother during her pregnancy. This article would seem to point out that this may hold true for the patient entering pregnancy with a normal birth weight. It's less likely to hold true for the woman who is obese when she becomes pregnant. It may be time for physicians caring for pregnant women to reconsider restricting weight gain to 25 lb, plus or minus 5 lb, to reduce the incidence of macrosomic infants.*

Pregnancy and Travel

Barry M, Bia F
JAMA 261:728–731, Feb 3, 1989 **2–2**

Pregnant women need not fear traveling if they are willing to take reasonable precautions. Any immunizations needed are best completed before conception but, in any case, the risk of acquiring a vaccine-preventable disease outweighs the risk of immunization. The fetus is not endangred by cabin pressures in modern jet planes. Anemia, especially sickle cell anemia, does pose a risk. The pregnant traveler must assiduously avoid contaminated water and food; antidiarrheal agents may be used, but prophylactic antibiotics are to be avoided. Exercise is all right if it does not threaten the mother or fetus physiologically. Travel to areas endemic for chloroquine-resistant malaria is off limits for the pregnant woman. A final note: Belt up, even if it's a little uncomfortable.

▶ *Two of the most frequent questions that the obstetrician is asked is whether or not a patient can travel when pregnant, and what type of immunizations are necessary. This article does a very good job of answering those questions and, specifically, indicating what immunizations should be undertaken and what effects altitude may have on the pregnancy. It's recommended reading for any patient who wishes to travel, particularly abroad, when pregnant.*

Effects of Routine One-Stage Ultrasound Screening in Pregnancy: A Randomised Controlled Trial

Waldenstrom U, Axelsson O, Nilsson S, et al
Lancet 2:585–588, Sept 10, 1988 **2–3**

Can routine ultrasonography at 15 weeks' gestation be justified? Half of 5,000 women without clinical indications for screening at 12 weeks nevertheless were examined. Labor was induced less often in these women than in the unscreened control group. The earlier detection of twins did not alter the neonatal outcome. Low birth weight occurred significantly more often in the unscreened group, particularly when the mother smoked. A woman who sees her fetus on a scan might well be disposed to reduce her cigarette use! Although screening at 15 weeks does not lower the total number of scans done in pregnancy, it does reduce the rate of induction. This probably is a result of improved dating.

▶ *Ultrasound has become so sophisticated and so frequently used that hardly a pregnancy goes by, unless the woman has had no prenatal care, in which an ultrasound is not performed. The question is whether routine ultrasound is cost effective. This article would seem to indicate that there are certain benefits associated with routine ultrasound such as decreased frequency of the diagnosis of a postdate pregnancy and increased frequency of detection of twins, even though there was no detectable effect on the neonatal outcome among the twins. There is also a lower prematurity rate in screened patients. Similar studies are being conducted in the United States, and it will be interesting to see if they show the same efficacious results.*

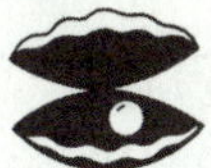

Almost every drug given the pregnant mother eventually resides in the fetus.

Fetal Bradycardia During Antepartum Testing: Further Observations

Druzin ML
J Reprod Med 34:47–51, January 1989 **2–4**

How does a policy of active intervention work out when, after 36 weeks' gestation, the fetal heart rate declines by 40 beats per minute or to less than 90 for a minute or longer? In a prospective series of 121 cases, with induction in the absence of obstetric contraindications, no fetal deaths occurred. The only neonatal death occurred in an infant with erythroblastosis fetalis. In this series, a nonreactive nonstress test predicted a low 5-minute Apgar score. Variable decelerations during labor, a cord compression pattern, were more frequent than the late decelerations of uteroplacental insufficiency. As long as lung maturity is confirmed, fetal bradycardia should prompt induction of labor. If lung maturity is in question, continuous electronic monitoring for 12–24 hours with daily testing for 3–4 days is the best course to follow.

▸ *One of the most bothersome things to a physician treating a pregnant patient is the onset of bradycardia during antepartum fetal heart rate testing. This study points out, as did an earlier study by Moburg et al.* (Obstet Gynecol *64:60, 1984), that this type of bradycardia is not totally benign for the fetus, and that, if it does occur in the presence of fetal maturity, wisdom dictates that the fetus be delivered. If there is fetal immaturity, the fetus should be monitored on a daily basis and ultrasound used to make certain that there is not oligohydramnios, resulting in umbilical cord compression.*

The Safety and Efficacy of Chorionic Villus Sampling for Early Prenatal Diagnosis of Cytogenetic Abnormalities

Rhoads GG, Jackson LG, Schlesselman SE, et al
N Engl J Med 320:609–617, March 9, 1989 **2–5**

The new alternative to amniocentesis: Take tissue for genetic study from the developing placenta using a catheter placed transcervically under ultrasound guidance. Nearly 2,300 women had chorionic villus sampling (CVS), chiefly because of age 33 or older; 670 others had amniocentesis at 16 weeks' gestation. Fewer than 1% of the women having CVS later underwent amniocentesis because of an uncertain diagnosis. There were no incorrect determinations of sex, and major trisomies were identified consistently. Total losses after CVS exceeded those in the amniocentesis group by less than 1%. No serious maternal infections occurred in either group, or in another 2,000 women having CVS. This is a generally safe and efficient means of prenatal diagnosis.

▸ *This multicenter trial indicates that there is a small increased risk, less than 1%, associated with CVS; however, the advantages—early diagnosis and a much easier abortion at 10–12 weeks of gestation if that's elected, as compared to 16–18 weeks—would seem to me to far outweigh this slight disadvantage.*

A Laparoscopic Approach Can Be Applied to Most Cases of Ectopic Pregnancy

Silva PD
Obstet Gynecol 72:944–947, December 1988 **2–6**

The latest of the many new approaches to ectopic pregnancy is laparoscopic electrosurgery. The proximal tube and mesosalpinx are electrocoagulated and cut or, if the oviduct is unruptured and future fertility is desired, salpingostomy is done with the unipolar needle point or knife cautery and vasopressin is injected into the mesosalpinx. Twenty-two patients were effectively treated, with an average added blood loss of 30 mL. Patients were hospitalized only 1 day on average and were able to return to work within 1–2 weeks. Most unselected patients with ectopic pregnancy can be managed laparoscopically at low cost and with low morbidity. The contraindications: hemodynamic instability, abdominal gestation, or an invisible mesosalpinx.

► *Laparoscopy has certainly achieved widespread use in the past decade, permitting patients to have much less extensive surgical procedures. This further development of laparoscopy—the successful treatment of ectopic pregnancies through the laparoscope—can permit a much shorter hospitalization. Also, the results seem to be comparable to those of a full-scale laparotomy.*

Incidence of Early Loss of Pregnancy

Wilcox AJ, Weinberg CR, O'Connor JF, et al
N Engl J Med 19:189–194, July 28, 1988 **2–7**

Healthy couples who regularly have unprotected intercourse have a 25% to 30% chance of conceiving in a given cycle. When pregnancy is not recognized, how often is this because of an early loss? This question was asked using a highly sensitive immunoradiometric assay for human chorionic gonadotropin in 221 healthy women who tried to conceive in 700 menstrual cycles. Of about 200 pregnancies detected, 22% ended before they were clinically apparent. The women were normally fertile: all but 5% of 40 with clinically inapparent early pregnancy losses conceived again within 2 years. The overall rate of pregnancy loss, including clinical spontaneous abortions, was 31%, and about two thirds were early losses.

► *Reported pregnancy loss during the first trimester has varied from 10% to 30%, the loss rate being directly proportional to the sophistication with which one diagnoses pregnancy. These figures become important when one compares the success of an artificial method such as in vitro fertilization to spontaneous pregnancy.*

Karyotypes of 1,142 Couples With Recurrent Abortion

Portnoï M-F, Joye N, Van den Akuer J, et al
Obstet Gynecol 72:31–34, July 1988 **2–8**

Major chromosomal rearrangements occurred in 5% of this large series and chromosomal variants in 3.5%. The rate of rearrangement did not relate to the number of abortions in 770 couples with only first-trimester abortions. Cytogenetic abnormalities were most frequent—6.6%—in 255 couples with recurrent fetal wastage who also had at least 1 normal child. Thirty-four couples with a major chromosomal rearrangement subsequently had prenatal diagnosis, and no fetal abnormalities were found. Twenty-seven couples had normal gestations, and all of the infants had a normal phenotype.

▶ *Part of the standard work-up of a woman who has recurrent abortion is to karyotype both the prospective mother and father. This article demonstrates that a major chromosomal abnormality among these couples is a relative rarity—4.8% in this series—and that, further, the frequency of abnormal karyotyping does not correlate with the number of spontaneous abortions. Nevertheless, I believe it is worthwhile to karyotype those patients who have had 3 or more spontaneous abortions.*

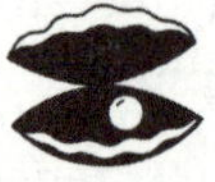

Significant amounts of endometriosis can be asymptomatic. Suspect it in the otherwise normal infertile couple.

A Randomized Study of Antibiotic Therapy in Idiopathic Preterm Labor

Morales WJ, Angel JL, O'Brien WF, et al
Obstet Gynecol 72:829–833, December 1988 **2–9**

Some preterm births not caused by obstetric complications or premature rupture of the membranes may reflect intrauterine or cervicovaginal infection. In a prospective study of 150 patients in labor at 21–34 weeks, 16 were found to have positive amniotic fluid cultures. Study of the placenta showed chorioamnionitis in 22 culture-negative patients. Treatment with either ampicillin or erythromycin for 10 days significantly delayed delivery. In women with negative cultures, colonization of the cervix with group B streptococcus or *Gardnerella vaginalis* increased the risk of prematurity, and the risk declined with ampicillin therapy. It may well be that antibiotic therapy combined with tocolysis is the best approach to idiopathic preterm labor.

▶ *McGregor* (Am J Obstet Gynecol *154:98, 1986) determined in a controlled study that patients at high risk for premature labor had a lower incidence of this when treated prophylactically with erythromycin. The present study would seem to carry that observation a step further, indicating that patients in preterm labor treated with erythromycin have a somewhat better result in terms of delay of delivery than those treated with placebo. The evidence is rapidly accumulating that a significant proportion of preterm labor is associated with infection in the amnion chorion or amniotic fluid.*

Evaluation of the New Amniostat-FLM Test for the Detection of Phosphatidylglycerol in Contaminated Fluids

Towers CV, Garike TJ
Am J Obstet Gynecol 160:298–303, February 1989 **2–10**

The new Amniostat-FLM slide test can detect as little as 0.5 μg of phosphatidylglycerol per milliliter of fluid (down from 2 μg/mL). In assessing 90 vaginal pool samples and contaminated amniocentesis samples, the findings agreed with those of 2-dimensional thin-layer chromatography in nearly 90% of cases. No hyaline membrane disease occurred when a test done within 72 hours of delivery was positive. The method is an ultrasensitive, simple, and rapid means of assessing fetal lung maturity.

▶ *Determining fetal lung maturity from vaginal pool fluids and contaminated amniotic fluids has been difficult at best. Fortunately, phosphatidylglycerol is not influenced by contamination, either in the vaginal pool or by blood. This relatively simple test, which can be done quickly, yields a result that allows proper management of the patient with premature rupture of the membranes.*

Multicentre Randomised Clinical Trial of Chorion Villus Sampling and Amniocentesis: First Report

Canadian Collaborative CVS-Amniocentesis Clinical Trial Group
Lancet 1:1–6, Jan 7, 1989 **2–11**

Before introducing transcervical chorionic villus sampling (CVS) into Canada, a randomized trial was undertaken comparing it with amniocentesis in almost 2,800 women aged 35 or more. Sampling was done at 9–12 weeks' gestation, or amniocentesis at 15–17 weeks, to detect chromosomal abnormalities. Total losses were 7.6% after initial CVS and 7.0% after amniocentesis. Birth weights and the number of preterm births were comparable, but perinatal mortality was greater in the CVS group, especially in pregnancies of more than 28 weeks. Maternal morbidity was similar in the 2 groups. There were more problems in interpreting CVS samples, but, when indicated, amniocentesis clarified the situation. Overall, these findings should serve to reassure women about the safety of first-trimester CVS.

▶ *Chorionic villus sampling gives a much earlier diagnosis of genetic abnormalities. The fear was that there would be increased pregnancy loss associated with the procedure. This large trial demonstrates that pregnancy loss, in comparison with amniocentesis, is minimal, the difference being less than 1% at best.*

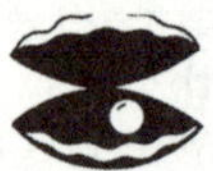

A midpelvic forceps delivery of the vertex of a large fetus is courting shoulder dystocia.

A Case-Control Study of Chorioamnionic Infection and Histologic Chorioamnionitis in Prematurity

Hillier SL, Martius J, Krohn M, et al
N Engl J Med 319:972–978, Oct 13, 1988 **2–12**

In a case-control study of nearly 100 women, chorioamnionic organisms were present in 23 of 38 (61%) who delivered before 37 weeks' gestation and in 12 of 56 (21%) who delivered at term. About half of the isolates from women who delivered prematurely were *Ureaplasma urealyticum* and another fourth were *Gardnerella vaginalis*, but recovery of any organism was closely associated with histologic changes of chorioamnionitis as well as with bacterial vaginosis. Women delivering earliest were the most likely to have infection. Premature delivery remained related to both chorioamnionic organisms and chorioamnionitis after controlling for demographic and obstetric factors. Because even a small reduction in the rate of prematurity would be most salutary, controlled trials of antimicrobial therapy are warranted.

▶ *Chorioamnionitis in pregnancy is an extremely common etiology of preterm delivery. The organisms most frequently mentioned are* Escherichia coli *and beta-hemolytic streptococci, and, occasionally, mycoplasma. This article points out that the 2 most common organisms isolated from the chorioamnion were* U. urealyticum *(47%) and* G. vaginalis *(26%). Thus, if we are going to reduce the incidence of preterm birth attributable to this chorioamnionitis we must start treating with antibiotics that will successfully eradicate* U. urealyticum *and* G. vaginalis. *This would include erythromycin and gentamicin.*

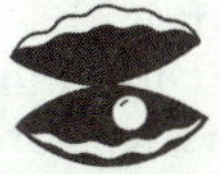

If the mother had preeclampsia, watch out for it in her daughter.

The Role of Infection in the Etiology of Preterm Birth

Toth M, Witkin SS, Ledger W, et al
Obstet Gynecol 71:723–726, May 1988 **2–13**

Does infection regularly precede preterm birth or premature rupture of the membranes? In about 200 unselected women, preterm birth related closely to both a history of pelvic inflammatory disease (PID) and previous use of an intrauterine device (IUD). Past PID as well as the presence of IgG antisperm antibody predicted the occurrence of amnionitis. The factors most accurately predicting the end of pregnancy before 37 weeks were a combined history of PID/IUD use and maternal age. Premature membrane rupture occurred more often in women having multiple sex partners. Possibly, previous genital tract infection is the first link in the chain: Asymptomatic colonization of the uterus—clinical infection when host defenses are altered in pregnancy—invasion of the membranes, placenta, and amniotic fluid could lead to pregnancy loss.

▶ *This paper looks at some of the interesting precursors that one might associate with infection and relates them to preterm labor. These precursors include a history of PID and multiple sexual partners, both of which were strongly associated with the history of premature labor. Preterm labor is one of the most significant problems in obstetrics today, accounting for substantial perinatal mortality, perinatal morbidity, and cost to the health care system. If the diagnosis is made early in labor, there is good evidence in multiple studies that tocolysis can be effective in reducing this complication. Thus any predictive factors for preterm labor assume extreme importance.*

Maternal and Neonatal Transport: Results of a National Collaborative Survey of Preterm and Very Low Birth Weight Infants in the Netherlands

Kollée LA, Verloove-Vanhorick SP, Verwey RA, et al
Obstet Gynecol 72:729–732, November 1988 **2–14**

A Dutch series of 1,340 infants born at 32 weeks' gestation or earlier served to compare transport of the mother or newborn infant to a university center with delivery or neonatal care at a local or regional hospital. Infants born after the mother was taken to a center had a significantly lower mortality risk. In addition, respiratory distress syndrome was less frequent. More infants taken to centers for neonatal care survived, but the difference was not significant. Delivery at a tertiary prenatal center indeed offers the best chance for early preterm infants. Regionalized prenatal care with maternal transport might reduce the number of neonates transported without increasing total admissions to neonatal intensive care.

▶ *The uterus is still the best incubator and the best transport mechanism for the immature fetus. The physician must be aware of early signs of impending premature labor and make the patient aware of those signs as well. The patient who is in premature labor should be taken as quickly as possible to a hospital that can provide the most sophisticated care should that premature infant be delivered. This is particularly important for those infants weighing less than 1,500 g or are less than 32 weeks of gestation.*

Morbidity of Very Low Birthweight Infants at Corrected Age of Two Years in a Geographically Defined Population: Report From Project on Preterm and Small for Gestational Age Infants in the Netherlands

van Zeben-van der Aa TM, Verloove-Vanhorick SP, Brand R, et al
Lancet 1:253–255, Feb 4, 1989 **2–15**

Of a thousand infants born before 32 completed weeks of gestation or weighing less than 1,500 g, 59 had a major handicap at age 2 years and 111 others had a minor handicap. Mortality in the first 2 years of life was 28%, and it related to gestational age. Handicaps, in contrast, were unrelated to gestational age and birth weight. More than half of the handicapped children had a central motor deficit, usually cerebral palsy. Those with a major degree of handicap often were mentally retarded as well. Possible risk factors for handicap at age 2 years included the obstetric history, fetal presentation, mode of delivery, socioeconomic status, and the neonatal occurrence of respiratory distress syndrome or intracranial bleeding.

▶ *As the obstetrician delivers smaller and smaller babies, and the pediatrician is successful in maintaining life in those babies, one of the principal worries is the subsequent neurologic development of these very-low-birth-weight infants. Fifteen or more years ago, 80% of such infants weighing less than 1,500 g had some neurologic handicap. It's encouraging to see that, at the present time, this incidence has fallen to less than 10% in most reported series.*

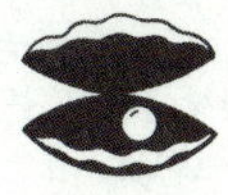

Headache, visual disturbances, and abdominal pain are all signs mandating hospital admission in any pregnant patient with blood pressure elevation or proteinuria.

The Differential Effect of Prenatal Care on the Incidence of Low Birth Weight Among Blacks and Whites in a Prepaid Health Care Plan

Murray JL, Bernfield M
N Engl J Med 319:1385–1391, Nov 24, 1988 **2–16**

Because improved prenatal care improves birth outcomes, barriers to receiving care could explain some of the difference in outcomes between blacks and whites. In a series of almost 32,000 deliveries, black mothers used prenatal care less than whites and had more low-birth-weight infants. This, however, accounted for less than 15% of the difference in low-weight infants. Higher levels of prenatal care had a greater effect on birth weights, especially very low birth weights, in the blacks than in whites. Apparently, blacks use prepaid prenatal services less than whites do, but they benefit more from such care. If we knew more about what determines the use of prenatal care the findings might be most salutary.

▶ *It has been reported for many years that the incidence of low-birth-weight and very-low-birth-weight infants is significantly higher in black, as compared to white, newborns. It was assumed that this was because of the lower incidence of prenatal care in the black population, which seems to be borne out in this article. The use of prenatal care is extremely beneficial for both populations, particularly the black population, and every effort should be made to encourage all mothers to seek prenatal care. Good prenatal care is one of the ways to cut down the overall cost of pregnancy. A large number of prenatal visits can be accommodated at the cost of an infant's single-day stay in the newborn intensive care unit.*

Traumatic Injury in Large-for-Date Infants

Wikström I, Axelsson O, Bergström R, et al
Acta Obstet Gynecol Scand 67:259–264, 1988 **2–17**

Delivery is a risky business for the excessively large fetus. When 500 infants weighing at least 4,500 g at term (3% of all infants delivered in 5 years) were compared with a normal-weight group, traumatic injuries were found in 8% of the large infants and in fewer than 1% of control infants. The fractured clavicle was most frequent, but 4 large infants had a broken humerus and 12 had brachial plexus injuries; 6 had multiple injuries. In addition to birth weight, factors such as postterm pregnancy, forceps delivery, and vacuum extraction all increased the risk of injury. Both high birth weight and postterm pregnancy correlated with a low 1-minute Apgar score. Large infants deserve as much obstetric attention as do the small ones.

▶ *Even though large-for-date infants (weighing more than 4,500 g) comprise a relatively small proportion of the total number of deliveries, they account for a significant portion of traumatic injuries, particularly Erbs palsy associated with shoulder dystocia. Many factors can alert the physician to this possibility, such as maternal diabetes, excessive weight gain in a woman of normal prepregnancy weight, and a history of previous macrosomic children. However, all diagnostic modalities must be used, including estimated fetal weight, progress of labor (i.e., slow progress through the birth canal in descent), and ultrasonic estimation of fetal weight to predict a large-for-date infant. If an infant is predicted as weighing more than 4,500 g, cesarean section is the preferential route of delivery.*

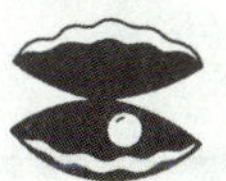

Late deceleration of the fetal heart rate indicates fetal hypoxia, and variable deceleration indicates cord compression. Thus the fetus with moderate or severe deceleration, or any latent celeration, must be evaluated carefully for the possibility of immediate delivery.

Severe Intra-Uterine Growth Retardation: Obstetrical Management and Follow Up Studies in Children Born Between 1970 and 1985

Schauseil-Zipf U, Hamm W, Stenzel B, et al
Eur J Obs Gynecol Reprod Biol 30:1–9, January 1989 **2–18**

Severe intrauterine growth retardation, i.e., a birth weight below the third percentile, occurred in 1.5% of infants born between 1970 and 1975 and in 1.1% in the following 10-year period. Comparing these 145 and 118 infants, premature delivery was twice as frequent in the later period. The rate of perinatal asphyxia in premature children declined, but perinatal mortality rose nevertheless because of more infants weighing less than 1,000 g. Excluding these very small infants, the perinatal mortality rate was between 2% and 3% in both periods. Cesarean deliveries more than doubled during the review period. Development was delayed in up to a third of infants, and about the same proportion had neurologic sequelae, mostly of mild degree. Term and premature infants followed a similar course. Improvements in the care of very-low-birth-weight infants in recent years provide some reason to be optimistic.

▶ *Management of the infant who demonstrates uterine growth retardation is always a dilemma for the obstetrician. In symmetric intrauterine growth retardation, it is important that one rule out severe congenital malformations and chromosomal defects. This can be done by amniotic fluid karyotyping as well as with level 3 ultrasound. The asymmetric intrauterine growth retarded child, although not manifesting any signs of intrauterine hypoxia, may remain in utero until fetal lung maturity is gained. Once lung maturity is achieved and there is no evidence of further growth, even though the fetus is not hypoxic it is probably best delivered.*

Cocaine Abuse During Pregnancy: Maternal and Fetal Implications

Little BB, Snell LM, Klein VR, et al
Obstet Gynecol 73:157–160, February 1989 **2–19**

What actually happens when mother is a cocaine user? Comparing 50 abusers with 100 unexposed women and their infants confirmed prevailing fears: Significantly more cocaine users had preterm labor, and more of the infants had complications at birth. In addition, these infants were lighter than the controls, and they had an excess of congenital cardiac anomalies. To show how tricky it can be to draw conclusions from studies such as this, many of the cocaine abusers smoked, but this itself did not relate to low birth weight. The anorectic effect of cocaine may have masked the effect of cigarette smoking.

▶ *Cocaine abuse is ever increasing in the United States. We know that it is associated with a significantly greater incidence of preterm labor and a higher incidence of infants in distress at delivery, with meconium staining of the amniotic fluid and tachycardia. This article also reports an excess incidence of congenital cardiac anomalies. This type of information needs to be made relatively available to all patients during pregnancy, because too many think that cocaine is a relatively innocuous recreational drug.*

Mother-to-Child Transmission of HIV Infection

The European Collaborative Study
Lancet 2:1039–1043, Nov 5, 1988 **2–20**

Of 271 children of human immunodeficiency virus (HIV)-infected mothers followed at 8 centers in Europe, 10 had acquired immunodeficiency syndrome (AIDS) or AIDS-related complex, all before age 9 months, and 5 of them have died. Twenty-two other children had clinical evidence of HIV infection; of the 12 with immunologic abnormalities, 9 were infected. The estimated rate of vertical transmission of infection in this series was 24%, but this probably is an underestimate. It is necessary to continue following children who become antibody negative, even if they are clinically well. The presence of nonspecific clinical features with a low T4:T8 ratio and hypergammaglobulinemia strongly suggests infection.

▶ *The increasing incidence of HIV infection among young reproductive mothers, predominantly in the intravenous drug user culture, increases the prevalence of infection in their unborn children. This study gives a much better prognosis than many others do, the latter indicating that 50% of the children born to HIV-positive mothers will contract AIDS. This study reports an estimated vertical transmission rate of 24%, which, if confirmed, represents a much better outlook for infants born to HIV-positive mothers.*

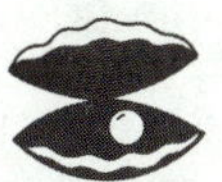

Start the normal pregnant patient on fetal kick counts at 32 weeks. Have her count the fetal kicks lying on her side for 2 hours after lunch or supper. (Four kicks in an hour is adequate.) This monitors the fetus and makes the mother rest.

The Postmenopausal Cystic Adnexal Mass: The Potential Role of Ultrasound in Conservative Management

Goldstein SR, Subramanyam B, Snyder JR, et al
Obstet Gynecol 73:8–10, January 1989 **2–21**

The pelvic examination is a subjective and not always very precise way of evaluating the adnexae. Perhaps ultrasound scanning can aid in the management of postmenopausal women with cystic lesions. Of 42 women with unilocular cystic lesions 5 cm or less in diameter, 26 were explored and all had benign cysts. One of the remaining 16 patients had an enlarging mass on serial sonography, done every 3–6 months, that proved to be a cystadenofibroma. Sonography can avoid surgery in postmenopausal women with small unilocular ovarian cysts.

▶ *There is an axiom of obstetrics that any postmenopausal woman with a mass had to have it removed immediately. With the advent of ultrasound, it has become apparent in several articles—one of which is abstracted above—that if the mass is cystic by ultrasound examination, it can be followed safely unless the mass is increasing in size or unless solid components are visualized.*

Calcitonin for Prevention of Postmenopausal Bone Loss

MacIntyre I, Stevenson JC, Whitehead MI, et al
Lancet 1:900–902, Apr 23, 1988 **2–22**

Because calcitonin inhibits osteoclasts, it might combat postmenopausal bone loss and thereby prevent vertebral fractures. In a 2-year study of 70 normal women, the effects of subcutaneous injections of human calcitonin 3 times weekly were compared with those of a combination of percutaneous estradiol and oral progesterone therapy, with both treatments, and with placebo. In doses of more than 250 μg weekly, calcitonin lowered vertebral bone loss as effectively as estradiol did. In addition, calcitonin reduced bone resorption more than bone formation, as was evident from urinary hydroxyproline and plasma bone-specific alkaline phosphatase estimates. As a practical matter, another means of using calcitonin—perhaps the intranasal route—is needed.

▶ *As stated earlier in reviews, bone loss is one of the principal problems in the postmenopausal patient. Some patients cannot take steroids to prevent that bone loss. This is an indication that calcitonin may be helpful in preventing this very devastating effect.*

Dietary Calcium and Risk of Hip Fracture: 14-Year Prospective Population Study

Holbrook TL, Barrett-Connor E, Wingard DL
Lancet 2:1046–1049, Nov 5, 1988 **2–23**

The costs of hip fracture in the United States exceed $6 billion annually, but the role of dietary calcium, a potentially controllable factor, remains uncertain. In a defined Caucasian population in southern California, 33 of about 1,000 individuals aged 50–79 years had hip fractures. The higher the dietary calcium intake (whether milligrams per day or per 1,000 kilocalories), the lower the age-adjusted risk of hip fracture. The association remained after adjusting for exercise, obesity, smoking, and alcohol intake. The message: Increased calcium intake protects against hip fracture. The question remains as to whether a higher intake after age 50 is effective, or whether protection reflects the calcium intake at ages 30–40 years, before peak bone mass is reached.

▶ *This article demonstrates the significance in the relationship between the intake of calcium and hip fracture. In all probability, the most significant factor accounting for hip fracture in postmenopausal women is the lack of estrogen. Nevertheless, the fact remains that many patients who start estrogen therapy in the menopausal period discontinue it for a variety of reasons, which include bleeding or simple failure to take the pill. Particularly in those patients, calcium supplementation would appear to be an important preventive measure in reducing the incidence of hip fracture.*

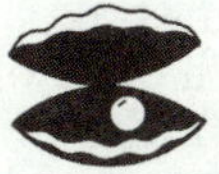

With amenorrhea and breast secretions, think pituitary prolactinoma.

Pituitary-Ovarian Responses to Nafarelin Testing in the Polycystic Ovary Syndrome

Barnes RB, Rosenfield RL, Burstein S, et al
N Engl J Med 320:559–565, March 2, 1989 **2–24**

Sixteen normal women, 5 normal men, and 8 women with polycystic ovary syndrome received 100 μg of nafarelin, a gonadotropin-releasing hormone agonist that stimulates pituitary and gonadal secretion. The affected women had responses similar to those of men: Early luteinizing hormone (LH) responses were greater than in normal women and peak follicle-stimulating hormone responses were lower. Androstenedione and 17α-hydroxyprogesterone levels were elevated in polycystic ovary syndrome even after pretreatment with dexamethasone to suppress adrenal function. These elevations did not occur in an additional patient with polycystic ovary syndrome caused by 3β-hydroxysteroid dehydrogenase deficiency. Responses to nafarelin are masculinized in women with polycystic ovary syndrome. A logical question: Is this a result of excessive LH secretion, or of an inherently masculinized theca-interstitial cell response to normal gonadotropin levels? Testing with nafarelin may help to distinguish polycystic ovary syndrome from other causes of hyperandrogenism.

▶ *Gonadotropin releasing hormone (GNRH) agonists have been very helpful in conditions such as uterine myomas and endometriosis, but this report suggests yet another area in which they may both prove to be a distinct benefit, i.e., polycystic ovarian syndrome. Patients with polycystic ovarian syndrome have a more masculinized pituitary and ovarian response to GNRH.*

Treatment of Premenstrual Mastalgia With Tamoxifen

Messinis IE, Lolis D
Acta Obstet Gynecol Scand 67:307–309, 1988 **2–25**

Mastalgia sometimes is the most distressing part of premenstrual syndrome. In 34 women with severe mastalgia, treatment with the antiestrogenic drug tamoxifen in a dose of 10 mg daily on cycle days 5–24 eliminated pain 89% of the time. The best part is that more than half of the women remained free of mastalgia a year after treatment ended. A placebo provided only slight and temporary relief.

Patients who have severe premenstrual mastalgia indeed have a difficult cross to bear. Tamoxifen, a weak estrogen, seems to be effective in treating these patients without causing significant side effects.

Clinical Trial of Naltrexone in Premenstrual Syndrome

Chuong CJ, Coulam CB, Bergstralh EJ, et al
Obstet Gynecol 72:332–336, September 1988 **2–26**

Beta-endorphin has a role in regulating the menstrual cycle. Possibly, withdrawal of opiate inhibition of biogenic amine systems in the luteal phase leads to rebound hyperactivity and, as a result, irritability, anxiety, and tension. The effect of the oral opiate antagonist naltrexone was assessed in 20 women with premenstrual syndrome. In most patients menstrual distress was substantially less when naltrexone was given from cycle day 9 to day 18 in a dose of 25 mg twice daily, compared with placebo. The menstrual pattern itself did not change, and toxicity never was so marked as to cause a patient to withdraw. The Menstrual Distress Questionnaire served to quantify symptoms in this trial.

▶ *A number of compounds have been tried without success in the management of this very difficult situation, premenstrual syndrome. This well-controlled, double-blind, placebo crossover study demonstrates the benefit of naltrexone, at least in some of these patients. Side effects were minimal. The effectiveness of this opiate antagonist seems to implicate the central nervous system in many aspects of premenstrual syndrome.*

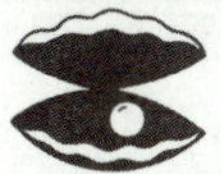

Absolutely regular menstrual cycles are seldom anovulatory.

Oral Contraceptives and the Hemostatic System

Farag AM, Bottoms SF, Mammen EF, et al
Obstet Gynecol 71:584–588, April 1988 **2–27**

Do oral contraceptives per se affect hemostasis? In comparing 130 pill users and 30 controls, direct markers of activated hemostasis such as fibrinopeptide A and platelet factor 4 were not increased. Plasminogen and prekallikrein levels were significantly higher in pill users, but levels of fibrinogen, antithrombin, and fibronectin were similar in the 2 groups. There was no overall increase in hypercoagulability in these oral contraceptive users. Perhaps more attention should be given to a family history of thromboembolism; among pill users, antithrombin levels decreased with a positive family history.

▶ *Every patient for whom we prescribe oral contraceptive therapy is told that she has a slightly increased risk of thromboembolic phenomena occurring. This does not necessarily seem to be the case, particularly if one takes into account a family history of hypercoagulability. It is always important to return to first principles: A proper history, including a good family history, is an extremely important adjunct to instructing the patient concerning her risk.*

A Prospective Study of Past Use of Oral Contraceptive Agents and Risk of Cardiovascular Diseases

Stampfer MJ, Willett WC, Colditz GA, et al
N Engl J Med 319:1313–1317, Nov 17, 1988 **2–28**

Current oral contraceptive use raises the risk of heart attack, especially in older women and smokers, but what about pill use in the past? Nearly 120,000 women aged 30–55 years were followed for 8 years. There was no evidence of an increased risk of cardiovascular disease in connection with past use of the pill, even prolonged use. This included major coronary artery disease, stroke, and death from all cardiovascular causes. The findings are generally reassuring to women who have used oral contraception but no longer do so.

▶ *Earlier studies with high-dose estrogen oral contraceptives would seem to indicate that there is an increased risk of cardiovascular disease, particularly stroke, and possibly coronary artery disease in those women taking high estrogen oral contraceptives over a long period of time. This study points out that this is not the case in those patients who have used the newer, low-dose estrogen oral contraceptives, even for a prolonged time.*

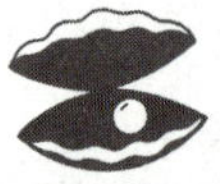

When a hysterectomy is necessary after age 45, discuss with the patient the pros and cons of prophylactic oophorectomy.

Oral Contraceptive Use and Malignancies of the Genital Tract: Results From the Royal College of General Practitioners' Oral Contraceptive Study

Beral V, Hannaford P, Kay C
Lancet 2:1331–1335, Dec 10, 1988 **2–29**

In a series of nearly 50,000 women, those who ever had used oral contraception had significantly more cervical cancers than those never using it. After correcting for many factors there was an excess of 41 in situ cancers and 8 invasive cancers per 100,000 woman-years of follow-up. After 10 years of pill use, women were 4 times more likely to have cervical cancer than never-users. Other uterine cancers and ovarian cancers were less frequent in ever-users of oral contraception. Because invasive cervical cancer can be prevented by screening, its early detection is especially important in women who have at any time used oral contraception.

▶ *The reported increased incidence in carcinoma of the cervix among those patients using oral contraceptive agents is indeed most worrisome, because oral contraceptive agents are the most effective means of birth control. In the past, the incidence of carcinoma of the cervix among oral contraceptive agent users has frequently been compared to the incidence in patients using some type of barrier method that is known to be protective. This article points out that the increase is mainly in in situ carcinoma, which can be cured completely if the patient is examined on a yearly basis with a thorough pelvic examination and a Papanicolaou smear.*

The Intrauterine Device and Pelvic Inflammatory Disease Revisited: New Results From the Women's Health Study

Lee NC, Rubin GL, Borucki R
Obstet Gynecol 72:1–6, July 1988 **2–30**

Only in the Women's Health Study, a hospital-based, case-control study done in the late 1970s, has the impact of marital status on the intrauterine device (IUD)-pelvic inflammatory disease (PID) relationship been considered. In comparing 650 women with PID and 2,500 hospitalized with nongynecologic disorders, the risk of PID related to IUD use did not correlate with a history of gonorrhea, the frequency of intercourse, or the number of recent sex partners. Among women with a single partner, IUD use increased the risk of PID in those who were previously or never married, but not in married or cohabiting women. The conclusion: Women at low risk of sexually transmitted infection need not fear using an IUD. The fact that the risk of PID is greatest shortly after insertion implicates nonsexual risk factors.

▸ *The IUD is an excellent contraceptive device associated with a very low pregnancy rate, both because of its inherent effectiveness and because one does not have to do anything actively to prevent pregnancy. One of the major fears developed after the use of the Dalkon Shield was a significant increase in PID associated with subsequent infertility. This article points out that those patients who are monogamous have almost no increase in PID when using the IUD.*

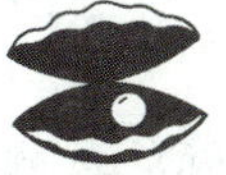

When colposcoping a patient, the tip of a suspicious lesion must be seen or conization is indicated.

Prognostic Variables in Treating Vaginismus

Scholl GM
Obstet Gynecol 72:231–235, August 1988 **2–31**

Vaginismus, a spastic reflex contraction of the perivaginal muscles, is by all means a major form of sexual dysfunction. Twenty-three women whose marriages were not consummated for this reason were taught relaxation techniques and encouraged to insert dilators of increasing size at home. Kegel exercises were prescribed as well and, if necessary, systematic desensitization was used. Twenty women were treated successfully; 3 however, whose circumvaginal muscles previously were divided, were unwilling to acknowledge that nothing was anatomically wrong. The key is for the patient to take responsibility for her own sexuality while, through using dilators, avoiding mere passive acquiescence with the sex act.

▶ *Sexual dysfunction can be a serious detriment to a successful marriage. Most sexual dysfunction can be treated adequately with good sexual counseling. The first step in this process is the determination that there is a sexual problem. Patients are frequently reluctant to talk about their sexual problems, thus a proper sexual history should be elicited from every patient.*

Acyclovir Suppression of Frequently Recurring Genital Herpes: Efficacy and Diminishing Need During Successive Years of Treatment

Straus SE, Croen KD, Sawyer MH, et al
JAMA 260:2227–2230, Oct 21, 1988 **2–32**

Fifty otherwise healthy patients with frequent recurrences of genital herpes for a year or longer participated in sequential trials of oral acyclovir therapy, 200 mg 3 times daily. Not only was the drug tolerated well, it was demonstrably effective. Eight patients required higher doses. The time to recurrent infection lengthened progressively after each course of treatment, and 10 patients remained well without further suppressive therapy. It would appear worthwhile to suspend treatment once a year to see what happens.

▶ *It's helpful to find that the long-term use of acyclovir can suppress frequently recurring genital herpes. We now know that acyclovir is rel-*

atively safe during pregnancy, so the disease could be suppressed in pregnant patients. The devastating effects of neonatal herpes (death or mental retardation) should be reduced to almost zero.

Clinical Manifestations of Vaginal Trichomoniasis

Wølner-Hanssen P, Krieger JN, Stevens CE, et al
JAMA 261:571–576, Jan 27, 1989 **2–33**

Culture or wet-mount studies demonstrated *Trichomonas* in 15% of about 800 women attending a sexually transmitted disease clinic. Many symptoms correlated with vaginal trichomoniasis: a yellow or purulent discharge, itching, vaginal/vulvar erythema, and the "strawberry cervix." These findings, although not highly sensitive, may be used to select patients for wet-mount examination. Either more frequent vaginal fluid cultures or immunofluorescence staining of vaginal fluid would improve the diagnosis and control of this infection.

▶ *Vaginal trichomoniasis is one of the most common infections of the female genital tract. It is easy to treat and easy to diagnose. It is particularly important that a wet mount be done on all patients complaining of vaginal discharge. In this age of expensive laboratory medicine, this test is inexpensive, specific, and beneficial to the patient.*

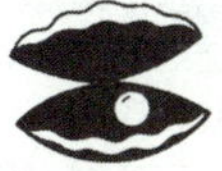

Cancer of the lung is the fastest growing cancer in young women. Get your patients to stop smoking, particularly if they are pregnant.

Diagnosis and Clinical Manifestations of Bacterial Vaginosis

Eschenbach DA, Hillier S, Critchlow C, et al
Am J Obstet Gynecol 158:819–828, April 1988 **2–34**

Of more than 600 women at a sexually transmitted disease clinic who did not have trichomoniasis, a third had bacterial vaginosis. The criteria: a homogeneous discharge with a pH of 4.7 or higher, an amine-like odor when mixing the discharge with 10% KOH, and clue cells comprising at least one fifth of all vaginal epithelial cells. Gram stain findings of bacterial vaginosis (*Gardnerella* and other bacterial morphological types without appreciable lactobacilli) correlated more closely with these criteria than did semiquantitative culture for *G. vaginalis*. At the same time, a positive Gram stain correlated with a clinical diagnosis of pelvic inflammatory disease. Bacterial vaginosis, an accepted risk factor for obstetric infection, may be a risk factor for pelvic inflammatory disease as well. Nevertheless, the authors reserve treatment for patients having symptoms and signs of the disease.

▶ *Bacterial vaginosis, nonspecific vaginitis, or* G. vaginalis *appears to be a condition that is being diagnosed with increased frequency among patients complaining of excess vaginal discharge. The presence of an alkaline pH, clue cells, and a fishy odor to the discharge after treatment with hydrogen peroxide should make this diagnosis for the physician. Gram stain may be very helpful in demonstrating the lunar-shaped* Mobiluncus*-type organisms frequently associated with this condition. Culture of* Gardnerella *may not be too helpful, because it is present in such a large proportion of the normal population.*

The Prognostic Importance of Steroid Receptors in Endometrial Carcinoma

Palmer DC, Muir IM, Alexander AI, et al
Obstet Gynecol 72:388–393, September 1988 **2–35**

How do steroid receptor values stack up against other prognostic factors in women with primary endometrial cancer? In a series of 350 patients, an estrogen receptor value of more than 70 fmol/mg of protein and a progesterone receptor value of more than 30 fmol were, along with age and stage of disease, independently related to survival. The presence of either receptor apparently confers a survival advantage, but the real predictive value derives from an estimate of how much receptor is present.

▶ *Tumors can be responsive to either estrogen or progesterone. This is extremely important information to have when treating the patient initially as well as for the long term. Those patients whose tumor is not dependent on progesterone or estrogen receptors can probably receive postmenopausal estrogen therapy that can control the potentially lethal side effects of ovarian failure such as osteoporosis and increased cardiovascular disease.*

Carcinoma of the Cervix in Young Females (35 Years, and Younger)

Chapman GW Jr, Abreo F, Thompson HE
Gynecol Oncol 31:430–434, November 1988 **2–36**

Is cervical cancer a distinct disease in younger women? Of 55 women aged 35 or less, 8 of them younger than 25 years, 35 had stage IB disease and 8 had stage IIIB or stage IV cancers. Radical hysterectomy with pelvic adenectomy, radiotherapy, and combined preoperative radiation and surgery all were used. Only 43% of women with stage IB disease were alive without disease after 5 years. None of the patients with stage IIIB or IV disease survived. The combination of young age and advanced cervical cancer may call for aggressive treatment, most especially, removal of diseased tissue after radiotherapy is completed.

▶ *Carcinoma of the cervix does occur in young women and may indeed have a more unfavorable prognosis, thus it is important that all patients be screened regularly for abnormal cervical cytology because carcinoma in situ is completely curable. The American Cancer Society has stated that the younger woman with 2 negative Papanicolaou (Pap) smears may be seen for Pap smears every 3 years instead of on a yearly basis. I think this recommendation should be modified significantly according to the patient's history. If the patient has begun intercourse at a young age or has had multiple sexual partners, I think she should have a Pap smear done at least yearly regardless of her age.*

Cigarette Smoking and Exposure to Passive Smoke Are Risk Factors for Cervical Cancer

Slattery ML, Robison LM, Schumen KL, et al
JAMA 261:1593–1598, March 17, 1989 **2–37**

As if there weren't enough risk factors for cervical cancer—and enough deadly effects of cigarette smoke! A population-based, case-control study in Utah, comprising 230 cases of carcinoma in situ and 35 invasive cancers, showed that personal smoking raised the corrected risk of cervical cancer by more than threefold. Exposure to smoke for at least 3 hours a day was nearly as dangerous, and this risk was especially great for women who themselves did not smoke.

▶ *The interesting association between cigarette smoking and an increased incidence of cervical cancer has been further extended to indicate that those patients who receive their cigarette smoke indirectly rather than directly also suffer the effects, not only of increased pulmonary cancer but also of increased cervical cancer. The enlightened industries that are insisting that there be no smoking in the workplace, as well as restaurants that have smoke-free areas and airplanes that are smoke free, will benefit a significant segment of the population.*

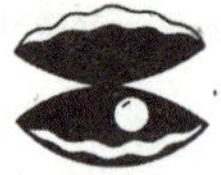

Endometrial polyps found at the cervix frequently hide endometrial carcinoma in the uterus.

Nylon Brush Improves Collection of Cervical Cytologic Specimens

Dotters DJ, Carney CN, Droegemueller W
Am J Obstet Gynecol 159:814–819, October 1988 **2–38**

A newly designed endocervical/ectocervical nylon brush for collecting Papanicolaou specimens was compared with the conventional cotton-tipped applicator plus wooden spatula in 400 women. The methods were equally effective for taking ectocervical specimens, but twice as many brush-collected endocervical smears contained more than 50 cells. Almost 20% of swab-and-spatula smears, but only 1% of brush samples, contained no endocervical cells. The brush seems useful, but perhaps not in pregnant women, many of whom had cervical bleeding.

▶ *One of the principal reasons for false negative cervical cytologic specimens is failure to obtain endocervical cells. Any Papanicolaou smear that does not contain endocervical cells should be suspect and should be repeated. The incidence of smears lacking endocervical cells could be reduced significantly using the cervical brush.*

The Cost-Effectiveness of Cervical Cancer Screening for Low-Income Elderly Women

Mandelblatt JS, Fahs MC
JAMA 259:2409–2413, Apr 22/29, 1988 **2–39**

This is the first economic analysis of cervical cancer screening for elderly low-income women. Papanicolaou testing was abnormal in 11 of 816 women aged 65 or older who received ongoing care at an urban municipal hospital clinic. Early detection of these cancers saved nearly $6,000 and 3.7 years of life for every 100 screening tests. If yearly medical costs were considered, the cost per year of life saved was about $3,000. Review of the findings from competing medical and economic viewpoints all confirmed that screening of these women is indeed cost effective. Programs such as this can save years of life and lots of money.

▶ *In these days of cost containment, each procedure should be examined to see if it is cost effective. Such an examination has been made for the Papanicolaou smear in a group of elderly women and, although the program cost $2,874 per year of life saved, carrying the analysis further could result in a favorable cost effectiveness ratio per screening. We need many more of these types of studies to evaluate our screening procedures.*

Preoperative Sonographic Evaluation of Endometrial Cancer

Cacciatore B, Lehtovirta P, Wahlström T, et al
Am J Obstet Gynecol 160:133–137, January 1989 **2–40**

Accurate clinical staging of endometrial cancer is not always possible. In 93 patients having preoperative sonography, uterine volumes were enlarged but did not correlate well with the extent of myometrial invasion. The volume of endometrial echoes did, however, correlate with myometrial invasion. Sonography was 91% accurate overall in predicting invasion; clinical staging was less than 80% accurate. Sonography is a good first-line imaging method in this setting. More complex and expensive tests such as magnetic resonance imaging may be reserved for patients with sonographic findings of deep or extrauterine disease.

▶ *The ability to diagnose the extent of invasion of endometrial cancer into the myometria can permit the surgeon to adequately plan the type of therapy to be undertaken. Should a wide radical hysterectomy be done? Should preoperative irradiation or postoperative irradiation be given? These are questions best answered on the pathologist's table. However, if sonographic evidence can accurately determine the depth of the invasion, it may allow preplanning rather than postplanning of therapy.*

Effect of Information Campaign by the Mass Media on Hysterectomy Rates

Domenighetti G, Luraschi P, Casabianca A, et al
Lancet 2:1470–1473, Dec 24/31, 1988 **2–41**

The number of hysterectomies done in a particular place at a given time appears to depend on many factors other than disease, including surgical bed density, payment systems, the surgeon's gender, and second-opinion programs. In a Swiss area where rates of hysterectomy and need for the operation were discussed in the mass media, operative rates fell by fully 25%. The rate in women aged 35–49 years declined by a third, as did the number of hysterectomies done annually by each gynecologist. In another area where no such information was presented publicly, hysterectomy rates rose slightly. Media campaigns do have the potential of helping physicians become better physicians.

▶ *Patient education needs to be done at all levels by the physician and through the mass media. Unfortunately, the mass media occasionally sensationalize certain aspects of medicine, and this can interfere substantially with proper individual patient management. The beneficial effect of mass media education can, on the other hand, be the reduction of unnecessary procedures, as this article points out. The only way we can combat the untoward side effects of mass media education is to confront the problems in our own profession first.*

PAP Class IIIA: A "Proliferating" Problem in Cervical Cytology

Vooijs GP, van der Graaf Y, de Schipper F
Eur J Obstet Gynecol Reprod Biol 29:219–226, November 1988 **2–42**

The class IIIA Papanicolaou smear denotes a range of lesions with minimal to moderate atypicality; they include atypical squamous metaplasia, slight or moderate dysplasia, and atypical repair reaction. Marked differences in the prevalence of dysplasia were apparent in 2 population-based cervical cancer screening programs in The Netherlands. In both series many severe lesions were found at follow-up after an initial finding of moderate dysplasia, but invasive cancers were infrequent. Invasive lesions were detected within 4 months after a class IIIA smear. The high prevalence of slight and moderate dysplasia and low rate of invasive disease suggest that not too much be done too early in following a class IIIA smear. In addition, even severe preinvasive epithelial changes sometimes regress.

▶ *Ever since Papanicolaou and Trout invented the Papanicolaou smear, the communication between pathologist and physician as to exactly what abnormal cells mean to the patient has been difficult. Rather than using a numerical categorization, I would prefer to use a nomenclature describing the pathologist's interpretation of the cells such as mild, moderate, or severe dysplasia, as this gives the physician a much better idea of what the follow-up or treatment should be.*

The National Cancer Institute Workshop has developed a system for reporting cervical cytology, the Bethesda System. This system is designed to give the pathologist the opportunity to report completely to the physician what is seen on the Papanicolaou smear. It includes a statement of the adequacy of the specimen for diagnostic evaluation, a general categorization of the diagnosis, and, finally, a descriptive diagnosis. The pathologist can include many of the previously used terms such as mild, moderate, or severe dysplasia carcinoma in situ, or CIN 1, 2, or 3, but will in addition include a diagnosis of squamous epithelial lesions, low grade or high grade. I would think that this system will give the referring physician a much better report of the cellular status of the smear.

3

Pediatrics

Lyme Disease: The Latest Great Imitator

Stechenberg BW

Pediatr Infect Dis J 7:402–409, June 1988 **3–1**

Because Lyme disease is endemic in some areas, pregnant women will be infected, and there have been adverse outcomes, although no definite link with anomalies is established. Along with the typical eruption of erythema chronicum migrans there can occur systemic symptoms such as neck stiffness and arthralgia. Myalgias, vomiting, sore throat, and regional adenopathy all may occur. Severe aseptic meningitis is frequent, but there also can be signs of brain dysfunction or encephalitis. As many as 10% of patients have facial palsy. Involvement of the heart can produce atrioventricular block, myopericarditis, or left ventricular dysfunction. Arthritis occurs, and commonly recurs, in many forms. Even transient conjunctivitis can be part of the picture.

▸ *It has been only 14 years since Lyme disease, caused by* Borrelia burgdorferi, *was first recognized. As with many disorders, the initial constellation of signs and symptoms associated with a particular disease entity are those that occur most frequently or that are most prominent in an epidemic situation. In the case of Lyme disease, the typical rash, known as erythema chronicum migrans, associated with joint swelling (arthritis), represented the hallmark of this disease as described in the medical literature. During the ensuing years it has become apparent that the spirochete that causes Lyme disease produces a wide variety of clinical symptoms and signs that are seen in disorders caused by other spirochetal organisms such as* Treponema pallidum *(syphilis), leptospires (leptospirosis), and* Spirillum minus *(rat bite fever). Subclinical Lyme disease can occur. In addition, upper respiratory infections, generalized myalgias, lymphadenopathy, or involvement of any organ system alone or in concert with others may occur. Physicians must include Lyme disease in the differential diagnosis in any patient who has been bitten by a tick, and they should consider the disorder in children without a history of tick bite who have fever of unknown origin, even in the absence of classic signs and symptoms of this disease.*

Lyme Disease: Acute Focal Meningoencephalitis in a Child

Feder HM Jr, Zalneraitis EL, Reik L Jr
Pediatrics 82:931–934, December 1988 **3–2**

Apart from meningitis and involvement of the cranial and spinal nerve roots, Lyme disease can involve the brain parenchyma. In a boy aged 7 who was infected by *Borrelia burgdorferi* an acute focal meningoencephalitis developed with hemiparesis and seizures. He recovered when treated with ampicillin and chloramphenicol but continues to require phenytoin. One in 10 patients with Lyme disease has some type of nervous system involvement. Direct invasion of the cerebrospinal fluid probably accounts for many of these cases. Ceftriaxone or chloramphenicol may work in the occasional patient who fails to respond to intravenous penicillin.

▶ *Meningitis has been described previously in patients with Lyme disease. The paper by Feder and associates represents the first report of involvement of the brain parenchyma itself in children with this disorder. This paper also documents the frequency of central nervous system (CNS) involvement in patients with Lyme disease and defines the relatively high incidence of such involvement (10%). Penicillin or ceftriaxone proved to be effective methods of treatment for CNS disease caused by* B. burgdorferi. *The frequency of CNS involvement probably has been overestimated, as many patients infected with* B. burgdorferi *experience subclinical infection.*

Treatment of Late Lyme Borreliosis: Randomized Comparison of Ceftriaxone and Penicillin

Dattwyler RJ, Halperin JJ, Volkman DJ, et al
Lancet 1:1191–1194, May 28, 1988 **3–3**

The key to treating Lyme borreliosis is to achieve good penetration of the tissues commonly infected, most notably the nervous system. A randomized trial of intravenous antibiotics compared 4 g of ceftriaxone with 24 million units of penicillin daily in 23 patients having clinically active late-stage Lyme disease. Although penicillin treatment failed in 5 of 10 patients, only 1 of the 13 given ceftriaxone had no response. Further experience with ceftriaxone in 31 patients, using doses of both 2 g and 4 g daily, confirmed its effectiveness. Three of 5 patients given steroids previously, however, failed to respond to ceftriaxone.

▶ *Penicillin has been recommended as the treatment of choice for all diseases caused by spirochetes. It is well known, however, that unless penicillin is provided early in the course of selected diseases caused by spirochetes such as leptospirosis, the drug has no discernible impact on either the duration of disease or its severity. The current study is of great interest in that the authors compared the use of ceftriaxone with penicillin in patients having late-stage Lyme disease. As anticipated from previous data, half of the patients treated with penicillin failed to respond. Most patients responded quite well to ceftriaxone, suggesting that it should be considered the drug of choice for patients with Lyme disease, particularly those whose diagnosis is made relatively late during the course of infection.*

Dexamethasone Therapy for Bacterial Meningitis: Results of Two Double-Blind, Placebo-Controlled Trials

Lebel MH, Freij BJ, Syrogiannopoulos GA, et al
N Engl J Med 319:964–971, Oct 13, 1988 **3–4**

Should dexamethasone be added to antibiotic therapy for infants and children with bacterial meningitis? Two hundred patients participated in prospective placebo-controlled studies of dexamethasone given in a dose of 0.15 mg/kg every 6 hours for 4 days. The antibiotic was cefuroxime or ceftriaxone. The response of glucose, protein, and lactate in the cerebrospinal fluid were more marked in steroid-treated patients. In addition, fever resolved more rapidly, and patients given steroid were less likely to have significant sensorineural hearing loss. The only death was that of a placebo recipient. The potential benefit from dexamethasone may outweigh its possible disadvantages.

▶ *Deafness occurs as a well-known sequela of bacterial meningitis. Lebel and associates claim that dexamethasone, provided for 4 days during the course of treatment of bacterial meningitis, may diminish the frequency of moderate or severe bilateral sensorineural hearing loss from 15.5% to 3.3%. Their data are applicable only to children with* Haemophilus influenzae *meningitis. Previous studies have documented that the frequency of bilateral severe sensorineural hearing loss in children with* H. influenzae *meningitis varies from 1.3% to 5.5% in those not given steroids. The reasons for the 15.5% incidence of hearing loss in the current study group in those who were not treated with steroids are unclear. This study has sparked considerable controversy, because all physicians would like to diminish to the greatest extent possible the frequency of sensorineural hearing loss in children with bacterial meningitis. There are many side effects of steroid therapy, however, some of which were experienced by patients in the current study. In an attempt to provide a definitive answer with regard to whether dexamethasone therapy can or cannot diminish the frequency of sensorineural hearing loss, a nationwide collaborative trial in which antibiotic therapy is provided with or without steroid administration is now being conducted.*

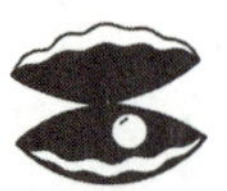

Four of the most important questions that a physician can ask in a pediatric history are pets, pica, travel, and consanguinity. Answers to these questions frequently provide insight into many infectious and noninfectious diseases.

Computed Tomography in Bacterial Meningitis of Childhood

Kline MW, Kaplan SL
Pediatr Infect Dis J 7:855–857, December 1988 **3–5**

Twenty-five of 85 children with bacterial meningitis had undergone computed tomography (CT) scanning of the head, most often because of fever, seizures, or evident increased intracranial pressure. All but 5 patients had abnormal findings, but in only 2 cases was the information of obvious clinical relevance. One of these patients had brain abscess and hydrocephalus, and the other had an occipital epidermoid cyst. Although not indicated for prolonged fever alone, CT may be helpful when there are focal neurologic findings, persistently positive cerebrospinal fluid cultures, or recurrent meningitis.

▶ *Computed tomography has been studied in children with bacterial meningitis during the past decade. This study documents that abnormal CT scans are the rule in such patients. A CT scan should not be performed on all patients with bacterial meningitis. It should be reserved for those who have persistent increased intracranial pressure after treatment (1) to document the possible occurrence of communicating or noncommunicating hydrocephalus; (2) to detect focal neurologic findings such as hemiparesis; or (3) to identify patients suspected of a parameningeal focus of infection such as brain abscess, subdural empyema, or intracranial epidural empyema.*

Current Therapy of Bacterial Sepsis and Meningitis in Infants and Children: A Poll of Directors of Programs in Pediatric Infectious Diseases

Word BM, Klein JO
Pediatr Infect Dis J 7:267–270, April 1988 **3–6**

Pediatric program directors were asked how they would treat presumed meningitis and bacterial sepsis in normal children. Most still favor standard penicillin/aminoglycoside therapy for newborn infants with meningitis. Infants a few weeks old usually receive ampicillin combined with cefotaxime. At 5 months ampicillin and chloramphenicol are used, but older children can be given ampicillin or penicillin G alone. How long to treat? The general rule is 1 week for *Neisseria meningitidis,* 10 days for *Haemophilus influenzae,* and 2 weeks for *Streptococcus pneumoniae.* Infants with presumed sepsis usually are given cefuroxime, whereas older children as often receive penicillin G or ampicillin.

▶ *Despite the advent of second- and third-generation cephalosporins that are presumably effective in the treatment of* H. influenzae, N. meningitidis, *and* S. pneumoniae, *these agents have not supplanted ampicillin and chloramphenicol in many centers as the treatment of choice for unknown septicemia or meningitis. I concur with the recommendations promulgated by most of the pediatric program directors. It is imperative that ampicillin be added to cefotaxime for children between 1 and 3 months of age because cefotaxime is not sufficient to treat* Listeria monocytogenes *or enterococci, which are frequent causes of disease in that age group. In children older than 3 months, ampicillin and chloramphenicol may be used, and cefotaxime alone would be a reasonable alternative regimen. I personally would avoid the use of cefuroxime because in infants with presumed septicemia the meninges may already have been seeded. At this time, cefuroxime is not considered a first-line drug for the treatment of meningitis caused by these common organisms, and either ampicillin, chloramphenicol, cefotaxime, or ceftriaxone would be preferred.*

Placebo-Controlled Trial of Two Acellular Pertussis Vaccines in Sweden: Protective Efficacy and Adverse Events

Ad Hoc Group for the Study of Pertussis Vaccines
Lancet 1:955–960, Apr 30, 1988 **3–7**

Because whole-cell pertussis vaccines can produce acute neurologic illness, 2 acellular vaccines were tested in 3,800 Swedish infants. One vaccine contained both lymphocytosis-promoting factor (LPF), detoxified by formaldehyde, and filamentous hemagglutinin. The other was an LPF-toxoid vaccine. A second dose was given after 7–13 weeks. Estimated efficacy during a 15-month follow-up was 69% for the 2-component vaccine and 54% for LPF-toxoid vaccine. Both vaccines were 80% protective against culture-proved whooping cough lasting for a month or longer. No vaccinated infant collapsed or had a hypotonic, hyporesponsive episode.

▶ *The currently used pertussis vaccine is the least immunogenic of all of the presently recommended immunizations for children. Efficacy has been estimated to be 70% at best. In addition, there are significant potential adverse consequences to the vaccine currently in use; however, the benefits from immunization in the young child far outweigh the risks. In an attempt to find a more immunogenic and less toxic vaccine, various acellular vaccines have been tested in recent years. In the study performed by the Ad Hoc Group for the Study of Pertussis Vaccines in Sweden, the 2 acellular pertussis vaccines had efficacy rates of 80% against culture-proved whooping cough, and no infant had hypotonic or hyporesponsive episodes. These data are somewhat disappointing in that it is unlikely that efficacy rates of 80% are sufficient to warrant a change in immunization policy with a recommendation to use 1 of the acellular vaccines at this time. The study group was far too small to document whether such potential complications of immunization such as vaccine-induced encephalopathy, which occurs in approximately 1 in 300,000 children, would or would not be a problem with the acellular vaccines studied.*

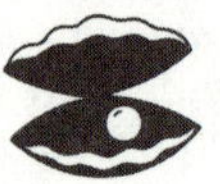

The male child with frequent urination and incessant thirst who is a descendant of the Ulster Scots should be evaluated for nephrogenic diabetes insipidus.

Risk of Sudden Infant Death Syndrome After Immunization With the Diphtheria-Tetanus-Pertussis Vaccine

Griffin MR, Ray WA, Livengood JR, et al
N Engl J Med 319:618–623, Sept 8, 1988 **3–8**

Reports of sudden infant deaths in temporal relation to diphtheria-tetanus-pertussis (DTP) immunization are an obvious concern, but these deaths peak at about age 2 months, the recommended time for the first immunization. In a cohort of 130,000 children with 109 deaths ascribed to sudden infant death syndrome, there was no increased risk of death after DTP immunization. This held true after controlling for age, gender, race, birth weight, and Medicaid enrollment. A large NIH study similarly indicates that immunization, most fortunately, does not make sudden infant deaths more likely to occur.

▶ *Many individuals and several network television programs have attempted to ascribe an increased incidence of sudden infant death syndrome to the administration of DTP vaccine. In particular, they have suggested that sudden infant death syndrome is specifically related to administration of the pertussis component of the vaccine. Several years ago there was an increased incidence of sudden infant death syndrome apparently in association with DTP immunization in the state of Tennessee. A very detailed investigation revealed that no cause and effect relationship could be established. The study by Griffin and associates, coupled with a large NIH study, clearly documents that sudden infant death syndrome* does not *result from the administration of DTP vaccine.*

Haemophilus B Polysaccharide Vaccine: Antibody Kinetics in 17- to 71-Month-Old Children

Ramsey KP, Popejoy LA, Jesse SW, et al
Am J Dis Child 143:28–30, January 1989 **3–9**

The serologic response to polysaccharide vaccine is less predictable and less prominent in younger children, but what is the course of induced antibodies over time? In about 200 children of varying ages, 90% of those given *Haemophilus* B polysaccharide vaccine at age 2 years or later had immune antibody levels after 3 weeks, but only 45% of those vaccinated at age 18 months had comparable titers. All children had significantly lower antibody levels after 6 months, and those vaccinated at an earlier age did not have any appreciable response at this time. Antibody kinetics may well be as important as the immediate response when deciding how to use a polysaccharide-based vaccine.

▶ *This study documents anew that the* H. influenzae *polysaccharide vaccine is not as effective when administered at 18 months of age as it is when administered at 2 years of age. The data provide support for the recommendation made by the Infectious Disease Committee of the American Academy of Pediatrics that* H. influenzae-*PRP vaccine no longer be administered. It should be replaced by* H. influenzae *PRP diphtheria conjugate vaccine, which can be administered at 18 months of age.*

Clinical and Immunologic Responses to the Capsular Polysaccharide of *Haemophilus influenzae* Type b Alone or Conjugated to Tetanus Toxoid in 18- to 23-Month-Old Children

Claesson BA, Trollfors B, Lagergard T, et al
J Pediatr 112:695–702, May 1988 **3–10**

Because *Haemophilus influenzae* type b capsular polysaccharide alone does not lead to protective antibody levels in young children, those at highest risk of *H. influenzae* meningitis, vaccine conjugates have been used. In 85 healthy children aged 18–23 months, unconjugated polysaccharide vaccine was compared with a saline-tetanus toxoid conjugate and with capsular polysaccharide adsorbed onto aluminum hydroxide. In contrast to the conjugates, no side effects occurred with unconjugated vaccine. Antibody levels produced by tetanus conjugate were tenfold higher than those achieved with the unconjugated vaccine. Responses of IgG1 and IgG2 were most prominent. The unconjugated capsular polysaccharide antibodies induced by vaccination were bactericidal in vitro.

▶ *This article documents that conjugate vaccines produce higher antibody titers than do unconjugated polysaccharide vaccines and should lead to greater protection against* H. influenzae *type b infection. The polyribose phosphate (PRP) vaccine licensed in 1985 for general use in the United States for prevention of* H. influenzae *has now been superseded. Current recommendations are to use the licensed PRP vaccine conjugated to diphtheria adjuvant. This newer vaccine produces higher antibody titers than the PRP vaccine does and is recommended for administration at 18 months of age rather than at 24 months. More recent data suggest that the diphtheria-PRP conjugate vaccine, when administered at 2, 4, and 6 months of age, may be effective even in very young children. Currently, other* H. influenzae *vaccines such as those described in this paper are being tested in the search for the ideal vaccine to use in the very young child who is at greatest risk for* H. influenzae *type b septicemia and meningitis.*

Reimmunization of Children Immunized at 18 Months of Age with *Haemophilus influenzae* type b Vaccine

Glade MP, Joffe LS, Brogden R, et al
J Pediatr 112:703–708, May 1988 **3–11**

Not enough is known about how long protection lasts after immunization with *Haemophilus influenzae* type b polyribosylribitol phosphate (PRP) capsular polysaccharide vaccine. Antibody responses to PRP given at age 3 years were compared in 25 healthy children who first received PRP alone at ages 17–19 months and 10 others given PRP plus diphtheria-tetanus-pertussis vaccine at this age. All but 5% of the children had post-vaccine anticapsular antibody levels of at least 1 μg/mL, compared with 70% of control children first given PRP at age 3 years. The mean antibody titer was about fourfold greater in children given 2 doses of vaccine. There were no serious local or systemic reactions to vaccination at age 3 years. It is reasonable to recommend revaccination of children first given PRP at age 18 months.

► *In an attempt to provide immunity to* H. influenzae *infection, several investigators have recommended using booster doses of PRP vaccine, because the antibody titer after an initial dose given to young children was either low or waned with time. This approach proved to be useful in the current study, but the use of PRP vaccine in 1, 2, or more doses has not been superseded by the use of the licensed PRP-diphtheria conjugate vaccine.*

Clinical Efficacy of a New, Enhanced-Potency, Inactivated Poliovirus Vaccine

Robertson SE, Traverso HP, Drucker JA, et al
Lancet 1:897–899, Apr 23, 1988 **3–12**

An outbreak of paralytic polio in Senegal, where the disease is endemic, gave an opportunity to evaluate an inactivated poliovirus vaccine of enhanced potency, N-IPV. A case-control study compared 89 patients who had residual paralysis with 384 matched controls. Children up to age 2 years were eligible to receive N-IPV in conjunction with diphtheria-tetanus-pertussis inoculation. The clinical efficacy for a single dose of N-IPV was only 36%, but 2 doses given 6 months apart were 89% effective. The outbreak of polio resulted mainly from failure to vaccinate, not vaccine failure.

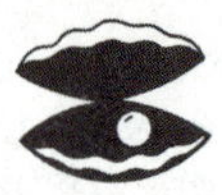

Evaluation of cerebrospinal fluid (CSF) for transferrin permits detection of a leak of CSF from the ventricular system through the nose or ear. An extra band of transferrin is located in the β_2 fraction as determined by protein electrophoresis of the CSF. This band is not noted in saliva, serum, tears, nasal secretions, or endolymph.

Live Attenuated Varicella Vaccine in Healthy 12- to 24-Month-Old Children

Johnson CE, Shurin PA, Fattlar D, et al
Pediatrics 81:512–518, April 1988 **3–13**

Live attenuated varicella vaccine was tried in about 250 seronegative children. No serious side effects occurred in the first 6 weeks after vaccination. Both infants and older children seroconverted at a rate of 95%, and more than 90% of converters retained antibody after a year. Mild disease developed in 2 of 24 children exposed to varicella. The Oka/Merck vaccine is safe, highly immunogenic, and protective against nearly all exposures to natural varicella for a year after vaccination.

▶ *Clinical trials of attenuated varicella vaccine have been carried out by numerous investigators in many countries within the past 5–10 years. The vaccine is already recommended for use in immunosuppressed individuals who are at high risk for varicella. There has been reluctance to approve the vaccine for general distribution because varicella virus remains latent forever in the host. Individuals who acquire varicella naturally (most of the population at the current time) are at risk for the subsequent development of herpes zoster. In the current climate of apprehension about medical malpractice liability, there has been some concern related to the liability of physicians and pharmaceutical companies who purposely give a vaccine to an individual to prevent one disease that, in turn, might produce another disease, namely, herpes zoster, many years later. Because there are many studies now documenting that the vaccine is safe, immunogenic, and protective in normal children, it may be licensed and recommended for general distribution within the next several years.*

Placebo-Controlled Trial of Varicella Vaccine Given With or After Measles-Mumps-Rubella Vaccine

Englund JA, Suarez CS, Kelly J, et al
J Pediatr 114:37–44, January 1989 **3–14**

One hundred healthy children aged 16 months, negative for varicella-zoster virus, received varicella vaccine, either at the same time as measles-mumps-rubella (MMR) vaccine or 6 weeks afterward. Nearly all of them had a serologic response to MMR vaccine; in turn, seroconversion to varicella vaccine was excellent and unaffected by the combined vaccine. Timing of the vaccinations did not influence the frequency of fever, rash eruption, systemic symptoms, or respiratory tract infection. A tetravalent MMR-V vaccine would be safe, immunogenic, and cost effective.

▶ *Varicella is one of the most common childhood disorders and has the highest degree of communicability from one nonimmune patient to another. Various varicella vaccine preparations have been tested and proven to be immunogenic in both normal and immunocompromised individuals. One of the issues that must be considered is the ease of administration and convenience with regard to providing for the patient. Even if the vaccine is approved, diminution in the incidence of varicella will be possible only if patient compliance with regard to vaccination is high. This report documents that varicella vaccine can be given concomitantly with MMR vaccine without affecting the safety or immunogenicity of either. We can look forward to the not too distant day when a tetravalent MMR and varicella vaccine becomes available.*

Effects of Dose and Strain of Vaccine on Success of Measles Vaccination of Infants Aged 4–5 Months

Whittle HC, Mann G, Eccles M, et al
Lancet 1:963–966, Apr 30, 1988 **3–15**

The measles virus still kills 2 million children each year and in some survivors causes blindness. The Schwarz vaccine is not sufficiently immunogenic in young infants, who are increasingly at risk of measles. Both a larger dose of the conventional Schwarz vaccine and the new Edmonston-Zagreb (E–Z) vaccine were evaluated. When 40,000 plaque-forming units of E–Z vaccine were given subcutaneously, a positive antibody response could be counted on. The same dose of Schwarz vaccine produced lower antibody levels. Even revaccination with either vaccine caused no adverse reactions. The E–Z vaccine may well provide the answer to protecting young infants in developing countries against measles. Global eradication of measles no longer is a fantasy.

▶ *A major outbreak of measles occurred in the United States during late 1988 and 1989 despite a current immunization policy that recommends use of measles vaccine (Schwarz or Moraten vaccine) in children at 15 months of age combined with rubella and mumps vaccine. In Houston, a city in which the largest outbreak occurred, there were more than 2,000 cases with 9 deaths, and more than 100 children and adults required ventilator management in a hospital because of primary measles viral pneumonia. Many young children became ill with measles before the recommended age of immunization, and adults and adolescents who had previously received Schwarz vaccine appeared not to have been completely protected. The possibility is exciting that a more effective vaccine is available for use in young children that might also provide long-lasting immunity. In the interim, the Advisory Committee on immunization practices has recommended a change in policy for the United States beginning immediately. The Committee now suggests the use of measles, mumps, rubella immunization at 12 months rather than at 15 months of age, with a second immunization for measles at the time of school entry.*

Patterns of Transmission in Measles Outbreaks in the United States, 1985–1986

Markowitz LE, Preblud SR, Orenstein WA, et al
N Engl J Med 320:75–81, Jan 12, 1989 **3–16**

Since the advent of measles vaccine in 1963 the disease is less than 2% as frequent as in earlier years. Of 150 outbreaks of 5 or more cases occurring in recent years, two thirds mainly involved school-aged children, and in a fourth of the outbreaks children younger than 5 years chiefly were affected. Only 27% of the measles in older children was thought to be preventable, but nearly half of the infections in preschool children could have been prevented. A twofold message is heard: Improve implementation of current strategies to eliminate measles, and consider further strategies such as selective or mass revaccination to limit transmission among highly vaccinated school-aged children. The costs may be high, but the effort can provide the impetus for a worldwide campaign to eradicate measles.

▶ *There have been more cases of measles in the United States during 1988 and 1989 than in any previous year in the past decade. Many infections have occurred in children immunized before 1980. Most outbreaks were thought to be related to the fact that vaccine produced before 1980 did not contain a stabilizer that permitted viability of the live attenuated virus under conditions of changing temperature that might exist in transport of the vaccine from the manufacturer to the site at which it would be administered. As noted in a previous comment, the Advisory Committee on Immunization Practices for the Centers for Disease Control has recommended that all children should receive measles, mumps, and rubella immunization at 12 months rather than at 15 months of age, and that a second dose of measles vaccine be administered immediately before entry into school. This is the first change in immunization strategy for measles that has been recommended since 1976.*

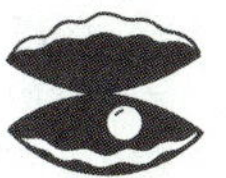

Children with fever of unknown origin frequently have common diseases with atypical presentations, or uncommon diseases with typical symptoms.

Efficacy of Oral *N*-Acetylcysteine in the Treatment of Acetaminophen Overdose: Analysis of the National Multicenter Study (1976 to 1985)

Smilkstein MJ, Knapp GL, Kulig KW, et al
N Engl J Med 319:1557–1562, Dec 15, 1988 **3–17**

After an overdose of acetaminophen, formation of a highly reactive intermediate can produce liver necrosis. *N*-acetylcysteine is an antidote that enhances glutathione stores as well as nontoxic sulfate conjugation. In 2,500 patients at risk, most of them females aged 10–30 years, an oral loading dose of 140 mg of *N*-acetylcysteine per kg was followed by 18 doses of 70 mg/kg at 4-hour intervals. Liver toxicity occurred in only 6% of patients probably at risk when treatment began within 10 hours of ingestion but in 25% of those treated at 10–24 hours. No patient treated within 16 hours died of acetaminophen poisoning.

► *Acetaminophen is the preferred therapy for increased body temperature in children. This drug is generally used rather than salicylates because salicylates impair blood clotting for a relatively extended period of time (in most cases this effect is not desired), and because salicylate toxicity has been a significant problem historically in children. The widespread use of acetaminophen has recently been associated with hepatotoxicity. The report by Smilkstein and associates is welcome because the authors document that* N-acetylcysteine *orally is a successful antidote against acetaminophen poisoning. When* N-acetylcysteine *treatment is given to patients with suspected acetaminophen overdose, it should be initiated within 8 hours of the event, but therapy is still indicated for 24 or more hours after ingestion.*

Chloroquine Treatment of Severe Malaria in Children: Pharmacokinetics, Toxicity, and New Dosage Recommendations

White NJ, Miller KD, Churchill FC, et al
N Engl J Med 319:1493–1500, Dec 8, 1988 **3–18**

Malaria remains a major cause of infant death in tropical lands, and chloroquine still is the best drug in much of the world. However, some have proposed that parenteral chloroquine no longer be used because of toxicity. Various regimens used in 58 Gambian children with severe falciparum malaria included 25 mg of chloroquine base per kg. Intramuscular or subcutaneous treatment with 5 mg/kg every 12 hours provided rapid drug absorption, but transient hypotension was frequent. With intermittent intravenous infusion, widely fluctuating drug levels indicated incomplete distribution. The answer seemed to be continuous infusion or smaller, more frequent injections. There certainly is no reason to abandon parenteral chloroquine therapy.

▶ *The authors of this paper indicate that malaria is still a major cause of infant death in tropical countries. It is important to recognize that congenital malaria and acquired malaria are still reported throughout the United States. Chloroquine has been the treatment of choice, but recent recommendations have suggested that its use be abandoned because of potential toxicity. As no other drug is superior to chloroquine against nonchloroquine-resistant strains of* Plasmodium, *various investigators have sought to determine whether changes in dosage or methods of administration might result in effective therapy and diminished toxicity. White and associates have shown definitively that continuous infusion of 0.83 mg of base per kg per hour for 30 hours, or smaller, more frequent intramuscular or subcutaneous injections of chloroquine (3.5 mg of base per kg per 6 hours), produce more constant blood concentrations with lower early peak levels and avoid adverse cardiovascular or neurologic effects. Chloroquine can be provided even in comatose children by nasogastric tube in an initial dose of 10 mg of base per kg. This report provides the basis for continuing the use of chloroquine in treatment of malaria, provided the drug is administered in the manner indicated in this paper.*

Bone Marrow Transplantation in Five Children With Sickle Cell Anemia

Vermylen C, Fernandez Robles E, Ninane J, et al
Lancet 1:1427–1428, June 25, 1988 **3–19**

Other severe hemoglobinopathies respond to marrow transplantation; why doesn't sickle cell anemia? Five black children from Zaire with severe sickle cell disease underwent allogeneic marrow transplantation in the first 10 years of life. They had frequent vaso-occlusive episodes but as yet no chronic organ damage. The marrow engrafted without major complications in 4 children. None of the children had a vaso-occlusive episode during a median follow-up of 10 months, and none has required blood transfusions. In 1 child autoimmune thrombocytopenia developed a year after marrow transplantation. Marrow grafting can cure young children with severe sickle cell anemia; it may be most suitable for those living where high-grade conventional care is unavailable.

▶ *Bone marrow transplantation has been used as a therapeutic modality for various hemoglobinopathies. The current study documents for the first time the possible efficacy of this modality of treatment for sickle cell anemia. Bone marrow transplantation is an extraordinarily expensive form of treatment, although this procedure would appear to be most useful in children living where appropriate ongoing care is not available. Unfortunately, it is unlikely that the procedure could be carried out effectively in areas in which the most sophisticated forms of medical care are not readily available.*

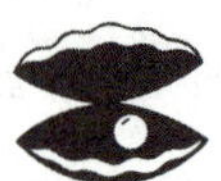

Radiopacities noted on plain radiography of the gastrointestinal tract in young children may be indicative of lead poisoning. They also may suggest, however, recent ingestion of Pepto-Bismol or a visit to the dentist (swallowed pieces of silver alloy fillings).

Prediction of Intravenous Theophylline Dosage Based on a Single, Nonsteady-State Concentration: A Clinical Study of Childhood Status Asthmaticus

Kurland G, Anderson DA, Mitsuoka JC, et al
Pediatrics 82:880–883, December 1988 **3–20**

I a single serum theophylline estimate sufficed to predict dosage, status asthmaticus could be rapidly controlled at a lower cost; at the same time, the asthmatic child would be spared multiple venipunctures. A hand-held calculator was used successfully to predict steady-state theophylline concentrations based on a single estimate made a few hours after hospital admission. An iterative program estimates the drug clearance needed to produce the measured drug concentration, and this in turn predicts the steady-state level. In 25 children with status asthmaticus, the predicted and measured steady-state levels differed by only 2 mg/L and toxic symptoms did not occur.

▶ *Theophylline is a drug that is widely used both intravenously and orally in the treatment of asthma in children. Its toxicity is well known, however, and in some cases can be devastating. Extremely high theophylline levels can be associated with seizures or cardiac arrest. Physicians who prescribe theophylline routinely measure the drug level to document that the dose produces a serum level in a therapeutic but nontoxic range. The current investigators report that, using a programmable hand-held calculator, they can predict steady-state theophylline concentrations and dosing requirements for children based on a minimum number of serum concentration determinations. Their results will be welcomed by all individuals interested in cost containment and even more so by the child who no longer must undergo repeated venipuncture.*

Home Intravenous Antibiotic Treatment in Cystic Fibrosis

Gilbert J, Robinson T, Littlewood JM
Arch Dis Child 63:512–517, 1988

3–21

The outlook for cystic fibrosis patients infected by *Pseudomonas aeruginosa* is much improved by intravenous antibiotic therapy, but this has required long and costly periods in hospital. A system of home treatment was designed in which a nurse served as liaison with the hospital. Forty courses of intravenous treatment, usually with tobramycin or ceftazidime, were given to 13 patients, lasting for 2 weeks on average. Body weight, lung function, and white cell counts all improved markedly. All of the families preferred home treatment, not surprisingly, because of better food, easier sleeping and exercising, and less interruption of education and work. Very substantial cost savings can be expected.

▶ *The respiratory tract of patients with cystic fibrosis is generally colonized by strains of* Pseudomonas *such as* Pseudomonas aeruginosa *and* Pseudomonas cepacia. *Until recently, attempts to diminish the frequency of such colonization and to treat* Pseudomonas *pneumonia required lengthy periods of hospitalization for treatment with aminoglycoside or third-generation cephalosporin antibiotics. The ability to treat these patients intravenously at home represents not only a step toward diminishing the cost of hospitalization but also toward improving the emotional well-being of these children. The development of third-generation cephalosporins effective in oral form against* Pseudomonas *will be of extraordinary benefit in the long-term management of these patients.*

The Effects of Physical Therapy on Cerebral Palsy: A Controlled Trial in Infants With Spastic Diplegia

Palmer FB, Shapiro BK, Wachtel RC, et al
N Engl J Med 318:803–808, March 31, 1988 **3–22**

Mandated programs of early intervention for handicapped infants often require a physical therapy component, but is this actually worthwhile? Fifty infants aged 1–2 years who had spastic diplegia were assigned to receive either a year of physical therapy or 6 months of infant stimulation followed by 6 months of physical therapy. The stimulation program involved cognitive, sensory, motor, and language activities of increasing complexity. Physical therapy was intended to improve expression of the postural responses of righting and equilibrium. Physical therapy offered no advantage over infant stimulation, whether in walking ability, occurrence of contractures, or need for bracing or orthopedic surgery. The moral: Any traditional intervention for developmentally disabled children should be viewed very critically; less costly measures may do just as well.

▶ *Many groups of investigators have developed extremely labor-intensive and costly programs that they claim will improve the outcome of infants with cerebral palsy and other developmental handicaps, including severe mental retardation. The paper by Palmer and associates documents that physical therapy offers no advantage over an infant stimulation program that involved cognitive, sensorimotor, and language activities. Additional studies of this type are clearly warranted because the field is fraught with emotional rather than practical responses to complex problems. Therapy appropriately should be based on facts derived from well-done clinical trials of different therapeutic modalities.*

Rett Syndrome: Natural History and Management

Moeschler JB, Charman CE, Berg SZ, et al
Pediatrics 82:1–10, July 1988 **3–23**

Eight females with Rett syndrome, a newly characterized developmental disorder that affects females exclusively, are added to the 600 such patients already described. Affected girls first have motor slowing and then obvious loss of acquired skills. Hand-wringing or hand-washing movements are typical at this stage; later, jerky, apraxic movements develop. There is an autistic affect—patients actually lose contact with their environment. Seizures may occur as dementia evolves and speech is lost. Eventually, the patient is left immobile, spastic, and wasted, bound to a wheelchair. Treatment is symptomatic and supportive, but merely making the diagnosis can help the parents.

▶ *Rett syndrome was first described in 1966 but not recognized readily until the mid-1980s. This disease, which appears to afflict female children, is characterized by deterioration in neurologic function after a period of normal development and is associated with seizures. To date, most investigators have focused on defining the clinical characteristics. Detailed investigations of the molecular basis of this syndrome are underway at the Rett Center at the Baylor College of Medicine in Houston. Recent unpublished data document definitively that Rett syndrome is an inherited disease. Investigations by Dr. Zoghbi are at a point at which the locus for the gene responsible for this syndrome should be identified within the next 12 months. This may lead to isolation of the gene and, ultimately, to gene replacement therapy in the next several years.*

Consensus: Management of Tuberculin-Positive Children Without Evidence of Disease

Grossman M, Hopewell PC, Jacobs RF, et al
Pediatr Infect Dis J 7:243–246, April 1988 **3–24**

The decline in tuberculosis (TB) in the United States has ceased, probably because of the increase of TB in persons with AIDS, in minorities, and in the homeless. An increased number of children are likely to become TB positive, especially in large cities. Experts were asked how to manage an asymptomatic tuberculin-positive child. All would give isoniazid for 6 or 9 months, depending on compliance, and half would add rifampin if the suspected contact had an isoniazid-resistant strain.

▶ *The incidence of TB has increased dramatically in the United States in the past several years. Grossman and associates suggest that this is possibly because of the increased risk of TB in persons with AIDS, in minorities, and in the homeless. It is important to point out that TB is found in children of all socioeconomic groups in all major urban areas at this time. In Houston, for example, 5.7% of all children entering elementary school were tuberculin positive. It is imperative that health departments in cities throughout the United States be aware of the risk of*

TB in the preschool population. Treatment with isoniazid for 6 to 9 months is ideal for the child who is a tuberculin converter. Routine screening for TB should be performed in children of school age in all cities in which the incidence of the disease exceeds 1%.

Identification of Human Herpesvirus-6 as a Causal Agent for Exanthem Subitum

Yamanishi K, Okuno T, Shiraki K, et al
Lancet 1:1065–1067, May 14, 1988 **3–25**

Exanthem subitum, or roseola, is a common infantile disease consisting of high fever and an eruption. Although the disease is usually benign, febrile seizures have occurred. A virus isolated from blood lymphocytes of 4 patients had morphological features of a herpesvirus. Convalescent sera seroconverted when tested against both the new viral antigen and herpesvirus-6 antigen. If viral infection occurs during infancy, seroepidemiologic studies should show a high antibody level that falls with age.

▸ *Roseola infantum (exanthem subitum) is a relatively benign common childhood disease. This disorder has been described in pediatric textbooks dating back to the late 1800s. Even in the most recent textbooks of pediatric infectious diseases, the disorder has been classified as one of presumed viral etiology. Studies documenting that herpesvirus type 6 is the cause of this disease now confirm previous suspicions and permit classification of roseola infantum as a disease of viral etiology. Isolation of the virus also permits development of specific tests for antibody to it that will be helpful in definitively documenting the presence of this infection in future generations.*

Use of Routine Viral Cultures at Delivery to Identify Neonates Exposed to Herpes Simplex Virus

Prober CG, Hensleigh PA, Boucher FD, et al
N Engl J Med 318:887–891, Apr 7, 1988 **3–26**

As genital herpes becomes more prevalent, neonatal herpes simplex virus (HSV) infections will increase. Viral culture specimens were obtained at 7,000 deliveries to learn whether such cultures would help identify infants at risk of neonatal infection. Herpes simplex virus type 2 was recovered in 14 deliveries. All of the mothers were asymptomatic, and only 1 had a history of genital herpes. However, 12 mothers had serologic evidence of past infection by HSV-2. The only infant with neonatal herpes was 1 of the 2 born to women with primary HSV infections. All women in labor should be asked about genital herpes and their external genitalia carefully examined. If lesions of genital herpes are found, cesarean section delivery is in order.

▶ *This article documents conclusively that most infants at risk of exposure to HSV at birth will not be identified if the physician is concerned only about asymptomatic shedding of virus in women who have a history of genital HSV infection. Most newborns exposed to asymptomatic maternal HSV infection at delivery currently cannot be identified. Infants born to women with genital HSV lesions should preferably be delivered by cesarean section; however, physicians caring for all newborns need to consider the possibility of neonatal HSV in the differential diagnosis of those who become ill during their early days of life, regardless of whether identifiable risk factors for HSV infection are present.*

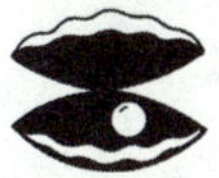

Calcification of the adrenal glands noted at birth is virtually a pathognomonic sign of Wolman disease.

Diarrheal Deaths in American Children: Are They Preventable?

Ho M-S, Glass RI, Pinsky PF, et al
JAMA 260:3281–3285, Dec 9, 1988 **3–27**

We all know that diarrhea is a very important cause of childhood deaths in developing countries—but in the United States? From 1973 through 1983 in this country, an average of 500 children aged 1 month to 4 years reportedly died of diarrhea. Deaths were most frequent in the winter, when rotaviral disease tends to occur. Black infants in the South were most vulnerable. A review of 40 deaths in Mississippi showed that diarrheal deaths were more likely when the mother was black, young, uneducated, unmarried, and received little prenatal care. Half of the deaths occurred after the child reached a medical facility. It may be that diarrheal deaths are "sentinal" events, pointing to deficient parental knowledge and inadequate medical care.

▶ *The authors of this article suggest that diarrheal deaths may be "sentinel" events pointing to deficient parental knowledge and inadequate medical care. Diarrhea is an extremely common illness in all children and adults. It may be caused by many different infectious and noninfectious disorders. Except under the most unusual conditions, death should never occur in a patient with diarrhea if there is appropriate knowledge about the use of fluid therapy. Although access to intravenous fluids can provide rapid correction of dehydration, in many children with diarrhea such access is not as important as the knowledge that fluid therapy can cure the dehydrated patient. Even in underdeveloped countries, severe diarrhea caused by cholera can be treated with an appropriate solution provided orally. Although massive volumes of fluid may be lost per rectum, fluid will be absorbed from the gastrointestinal tract if it is provided orally at a rate greater than that at which it is lost.*

Diseases Caused by the Human Parvovirus B19

Pattison JR
Arch Dis Child 63:1426–1427, December 1988 **3–28**

Infection by parvovirus B19 is very common worldwide. It may be wholly subclinical or clinically nonspecific, but the virus also causes erythema infectiosum, the fifth of 6 childhood exanthems to be described (hence the not unreasonable appellation, "fifth disease"). Joint involvement can occur in this disorder and may be the sole feature. The B19 virus infects red cell precursors in the marrow and limits erythropoiesis. As a result, patients with chronic hemolytic anemia may experience an aplastic crisis. If the transient but intense viremia occurs during pregnancy, virus can spread to the placenta and fetus, leading to abortion or, later in pregnancy, hydrops fetalis and possibly stillbirth.

▶ *The paper by Pattison documents the variability of human parvovirus B19 infection. It is the first paper clearly delineating that this infection may be subclinical or present as so-called fifth disease, which is characterized by an exanthematous rash. The author has also demonstrated for the first time that joint involvement may be the sole feature of this disease. This is one of the first papers clearly demonstrating that stillbirth, abortion, and hydrops fetalis may result from a transient but intense viremia that may occur in the pregnant woman. It suggests that pregnant women should be excluded from contact with children who are afflicted with erythema infectiosum.*

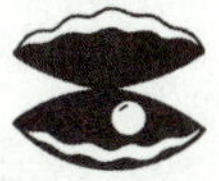

Extremely soft, pliable ears may be suggestive of chronic urinary protein loss and can be a sign suggestive of idiopathic nephrotic syndrome.

The Diagnosis of Group A, β-Hemolytic Streptococcal Pharyngitis in the Office Setting: Rapid Latex Test vs Throat Culture

Taubman B, Barroway RP, McGowen KL
Am J Dis Child 143:102–104, January 1989 **3–29**

It may be tempting to use the rapid latex agglutination text to diagnose group A β-hemolytic streptococcal pharyngitis in the office, but underdiagnosis is perilous in view of the rising incidence of acute rheumatic fever. When 2 experienced pediatricians independently evaluated almost 600 children, the latex test was nearly as sensitive and specific as throat culture in the office and false negative results were not significantly more frequent. The authors now use the latex test routinely—it is convenient and preferred by parents, and the results are available the same day.

▶ *There has been a great deal of discussion regarding the value of the rapid latex agglutination test for the diagnosis of group A β-hemolytic streptococcal pharyngitis in an office setting. In the study performed by Taubman and associates, the latex test was nearly as sensitive and specific as throat culture in the office setting, and the authors now use it routinely. The principal aim in treating group A β-hemolytic streptococcal pharyngitis is the prevention of rheumatic fever. The fact that the test is convenient and preferred by parents, with results available the same day, is not a sufficient indication for complete reliance on it if one is to achieve the ultimate objective. We recommend the use of this test in individuals suspected of having group A β-hemolytic streptococcal pharyngitis and the administration of penicillin to those whose tests are positive. When the latex test is negative, a throat culture to docu-*

ment definitively the presence or absence of group A β-hemolytic streptococci is warranted.

Partial Correction of the Phagocyte Defect in Patients With X-Linked Chronic Granulomatous Disease by Subcutaneous Interferon Gamma

Ezekowitz RAB, Dinauer MC, Jaffe HS, et al
N Engl J Med 319:146–151, July 21, 1988 **3–30**

In chronic granulatomous disease the phagocytes do not produce superoxide anion and as a result do not kill microbes efficiently. When 4 patients with the X-linked form of disease received 2 injections of recombinant interferon gamma, the granulocytes and monocytes produced 5 to 10 times more superoxide for more than 2 weeks. Granulocyte bactericidal activity increased, becoming normal in the 2 most responsive patients. This may well be yet another indication for using interferon.

▶ *There has been no truly effective means of diminishing the incidence of infection in patients with chronic granulomatous disease of childhood. This inherited disease, characterized by recurrent infections with* Staphyloccocus aureus *or enteric microorganisms, frequently leads to permanent disability or the patient's death. Prophylactic therapy with a sulfonamide drug on a continuous basis has been the only mechanism to potentially diminish the frequency of infections in these individuals. The current study provides definitive evidence that gamma interferon may be an effective means of preventing recurrent serious infections in these children.*

High-Dose Intravenous Gammaglobulin Therapy for Neonatal Autoimmune Thrombocytopenia

Ballin A, Andrew M, Ling E, et al
J Pediatr 112:789–792, May 1988 **3–31**

When a mother's antiplatelet antibodies pass to her fetus through the placenta, the infant can become severely thrombocytopenic and is then at risk of bleeding into the brain. Neither random platelet transfusions nor exchange transfusions are consistently helpful. But when 10 infants were given gamma globulin (IgG) intravenously, the platelet count at least doubled in 7 of them. Treatment was 1 gm of IgG per kg on 2 consecutive days. Five of 6 infants given steroids in addition to IgG had a good response. To assure hemostasis, some infants require repeated IgG treatment.

▶ *It has been only during the past 5 years that intravenous preparations of IgG have been available for use in children on an experimental basis. Ballin and associates document in their study that infants with severe thrombocytopenia related to transplacental passage of antiplatelet antibodies have improved their platelet counts when intravenous IgG is administered. Unfortunately, no therapeutic recommendations can be made based on the data available in this study, because infants were not randomized to IgG or placebo therapy. Prospective randomized studies of IgG vs. steroid therapy or placebo are required to establish the ideal treatment for thrombocytopenia. However, this study provides the basis for optimism that brain hemorrhage related to neonatal autoimmune thrombocytopenia can be prevented.*

Regulation of Genes for HLA Class II Antigens in Cell Lines From Patients With Severe Combined Immunodeficiency

de Préval C, Hadam MR, Mach B
N Engl J Med 318:1295–1300, May 19, 1988 **3–32**

In one form of congenital severe combined immunodeficiency (SCID) the HLA class II antigens, including HLA-DR antigens on peripheral blood lymphocytes, are absent. The products of HLA class II genes are cell-surface glycoproteins, which when absent impair the ability to mount a humoral immune response. As a result, the patient is subject to severe, often fatal infections, as well as severe malabsorption and failure to thrive. The genetic defect affects not only the B cell lineage, but also expression of class II genes in cells such as fibroblasts. Because the affected cells are unresponsive to gamma-interferon, patients with SCID will probably not respond to this lymphokine.

▶ *Our knowledge of the normal immune system has been derived historically from the study of patients with congenital immunodeficiency diseases. Patients with inability to produce immunoglobulins (B cell deficiency disease), those with impaired cellular immune function (T cell deficiency disease), and individuals with SCID (inability to react with either humoral or cellular immunity) are readily delineated today. Studies such as those by de Préval and associates show that there are many subclasses of both T, B, and severe combined immunodefi-*

ciency diseases that may not all respond to the same forms of therapy. It is only by defining these disorders at the molecular level that optimum methods for management and, ultimately, prevention of these disorders will be possible.

Impact of the Revised AIDS Case Definition on AIDS Reporting in San Francisco

Rutherford GW, Payne SF, Lemp GF
JAMA 259:2235, Apr 15, 1988 **3–33**

Recently, the CDC expanded the case definition of AIDS to include: (1) HIV encephalopathy; (2) HIV wasting syndrome; and (3) more opportunistic infections and malignancies. In a 4-month period in San Francisco the revised case definition increased AIDS reporting by almost 20%. Previous forecasts of the AIDS epidemic therefore will have to be revised upward and to a substantial degree. The most frequent new diagnoses are HIV encephalopathy, presumed toxoplasmosis, and presumed *Pneumocystis carinii* infection.

▶ *This report clearly suggests that former projections of the number of cases of pediatric AIDS in the United States will have to be revised upward. Previous definitions potentially may have underestimated the incidence of AIDS by at least 19%. Until 5 years ago, the leading cause of pediatric AIDS was blood transfusions contaminated with HIV. With the advent of widespread screening of blood transfusions for HIV, the number of pediatric cases related to transfusion has diminished markedly. Most children infected with AIDS today have contracted the disease congenitally from their mothers who (1) have either acquired the disease from a sexual partner, or (2) are intravenous abusers of various drugs.*

Live Virus Vaccines in Human Immunodeficiency Virus-Infected Children: A Retrospective Survey

McLaughlin M, Thomas P, Onorato I, et al
Pediatrics 82:229–233, August 1988 **3–34**

Live virus vaccines can have serious consequences in immunocompromised patients, and children infected with HIV sometimes are in this category. Of 221 HIV-positive children in New York City and New Jersey, 81% had received live oral polio vaccine and a third were given measles, mumps, and rubella vaccine. No child had atypical measles, paralytic polio, aseptic meningitis, or other serious event. During an 8-year period in these jurisdictions, no child with vaccine-associated illness had AIDS or a related illness.

▶ *Live viral vaccines are contraindicated for use in children with congenital forms of immunodeficiency diseases. Many individuals who are born immunodeficient, particularly those who have severe combined immunodeficiency disease or T cell deficiency disorders, have acquired overwhelming infection with the live viral vaccine provided for immunization. Often death has occurred. This study is particularly important, because an increasing number of children with AIDS are now seen in all major medical centers. The study documents that the general dictum found in all standard textbooks with regard to avoidance of live viral immunization in children with congenital immunodeficiency diseases is not necessarily applicable to those who have AIDS. This study forms the basis for the recommendation that, during the course of a measles epidemic, the risk of immunizing children with AIDS with live measles virus is less than the risk of permitting such children to acquire wild measles virus in the community.*

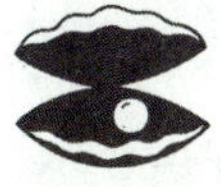

A child who persistently exudes an odor similar to that noted in a locker room may be afflicted with an inborn error of organic acid metabolism known as isovaleric acidemia.

Hearing Disorders in Children With Fetal Alcohol Syndrome: Findings From Case Reports

Church MW, Gerkin KP
Pediatrics 82:147–154, August 1988 **3–35**

Because craniofacial anomalies, as well as congenital cardiac and ocular defects, occur in children with fetal alcohol syndrome, it's reasonable to wonder whether hearing disorders are also prevalent in this group. In a series of 14 children, all but 1 had bilateral recurrent serous otitis media and 4 had clinically significant sensorineural hearing loss. Nearly a third of the patients had external ear anomalies. Receptive and expressive language delay was almost universal and sometimes was pronounced. It seems that prenatal alcohol exposure may account for more hearing and language disorders than previously thought. If this is recognized, early intervention may allow affected children to catch up intellectually with their peers.

▶ *Hearing disorders have not been recognized previously as an important consequence of fetal alcohol syndrome. The study by Church and Gerkin documents that prenatal alcohol exposure may account for a significant number of hearing and language disorders in this group of patients. The findings suggest that routine screening with brain stem evoked response audiometry should be performed as early in life as possible (before the child would normally begin to learn to speak). In individuals in whom hearing loss is suspected or documented, appropriate speech and language therapy should be initiated. The early detection of hearing disorders is essential if language therapy is expected to help the hearing impaired child.*

Infant Mortality Increase Despite High Access to Tertiary Care: An Evolving Relationship Among Infant Mortality, Health Care, and Socioeconomic Change

Wise PH, First LR, Lamb GA, et al
Pediatrics 81:542–548, April 1988 **3–36**

Regional increases in infant mortality are ascribed by some to economic hardship and lowered support of social programs. But others argue that such trends are subject to substantial random variation. A review of 422 infant deaths occurring in 1980–1983 in Boston, where there is high access to tertiary neonatal intensive care, showed an increase in mortality in 1982. The birth rate of infants weighing less than 1,500 g increased, as did mortality rates for both normal-weight infants and infants dying 1 to 12 months after birth. These increases were related to inadequate prenatal care. The adequacy of prenatal care did not affect mortality once an infant was born at a low weight.

▶ *The United States currently ranks eighteenth among all nations in infant mortality rates. This position relative to other industrialized countries may be viewed as highly unusual, as we have some of the most sophisticated facilities available for the care of the newborn infant and spend a greater percentage of our gross national product on health care than does any other industrialized nation. Reasons for the high infant mortality rate have been sought. The current article documents conclusively that, once a baby is born, there is a stable mortality rate for low-birth-weight infants that does not vary markedly between population groups. Far more important, however, is the increased death rate referable to lack of prenatal care. The relatively high infant mortality rate in the United States is largely associated with lack of access to appropriate prenatal care or the unwillingness of individuals to seek prenatal care when such care is available. Greater emphasis must be placed on the provision of appropriate prenatal care to all women before a decline in neonatal mortality rate will become apparent in the United States.*

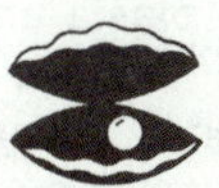

Ketones detected in urine obtained from a newborn infant in the first few days of life may be indicative of inborn errors of branched chain amino acids, organic acid disorders, or glycogen storage diseases types 1 and 2. Ketonuria in the first week of life rarely reflects starvation.

Ribavirin Administration to Infants Receiving Mechanical Ventilation

Outwater KM, Meissner HC, Peterson MB
Am J Dis Child 142:512–515, May 1988 **3–37**

Bronchiolitis caused by respiratory syncytial virus (RSV) poses a threat of severe respiratory impairment and even death to young infants and those with cardiopulmonary or immunologic disease. The synthetic nucleoside ribavirin improves arterial oxygen tension when given in aerosol form to normal infants with RSV infection. Twelve infants who were premature or had congenital heart disease or chronic lung disease had viral bronchiolitis or pneumonitis and required mechanical ventilation. Ribavarin solution was aerosolized and administered for 20 hours a day via a pressure-limited ventilator for 4 to 10 days. Eight patients had documented RSV infection. All 12 infants survived, and there were no adverse effects of treatment.

▶ *This article by Outwater and associates provides additional supporting evidence that aerosolized ribavirin is a safe, effective means of diminishing the frequency of complications and death in children with bronchiolitis who have preexisting congenital heart disease or chronic lung disease. Ribavirin therapy is expensive and difficult to deliver by the aerosol route. Sufficient data have accumulated to suggest that it should be recommended for children hospitalized with bronchiolitis who require mechanical ventilation, particularly those with underlying cardiac or pulmonary disease. The cost:risk benefit of using ribavirin therapy for routine bronchiolitis remains to be established.*

Task Force on Transcutaneous Oxygen Monitors: Report of Consensus Meeting, December 5 to 6, 1986

Pediatrics 83:122–126, January 1989 **3–38**

Oxygen is a lifesaver in the nursery. At the same time, however, it carries risks of bronchopulmonary dysplasia and retinopathy, thus there is a vital need to control oxygen therapy precisely. The transcutaneous oxygen monitor is accurate and clinically helpful, but the technique is not an easy one. Studies of infants in shock or hypothermia are suspect. Each time the electrode is applied, an arterial blood sample should be taken to estimate the actual arterial oxygen tension. Ideally, staff trained in applying the monitor and interpreting the findings will be available at all hours. If staff members provide good quality control and are aware of all possible sources of error, the transcutaneous oxygen monitor will be more of a blessing than a curse.

▸ *The use of oxygen is essential in most neonatal intensive care units managing the extremely premature infant. Even when the oxygen content of blood is monitored continuously, bronchopulmonary dysplasia and retinopathy may occur. The aim, however, is to diminish the frequency of these complications by using, if possible, an affective and noninvasive technique. This paper is recommended to all individuals who are interested in learning the details of just how transcutaneous monitoring should be performed. Of greatest import, it should be pointed out that this technique cannot be used to estimate Po_2 without periodically correlating this technique with arterial blood gas samples.*

Surfactant Replacement: A New Era With Many Challenges for Neonatal Medicine

Merritt TA, Hallman M
Am J Dis Child 142:1333–1339, December 1988 **3–39**

Exogenous surfactant offers the hope of saving infants, even very small ones, from respiratory distress syndrome (RDS).

The trials done to date, which of necessity included the most vulnerable infants, indicate that replacing surfactant is effective. Transient improvement is not good enough, however; there should be actual reductions in morbidity and mortality from RDS. It's hoped that an international multicenter trial will be done to compare the various surfactant preparations under study in different countries. It may well be that all infants expected to have RDS eventually will be candidates for this treatment.

▶ *Hyaline membrane disease was previously the leading cause of death in infants born prematurely. Many infants who previously would have had hyaline membrane disease are now born with normal lungs because their mothers are pretreated with steroids at or near the time of delivery when an extremely premature birth (before 36 weeks) is anticipated. In infants with hyaline membrane disease, artificial surfactant via a ventilator has proven to be beneficial in a number of different trials. The ultimate degree of reduction of morbidity or mortality from RDS in infants receiving surfactant is not known and requires initiation of a large, multicentered international trial.*

Surfactant Replacement Therapy: Impact on Hospital Charges for Premature Infants With Respiratory Distress Syndrome

Maniscalco WM, Kendig JW, Shapiro DL
Pediatrics 83:1–6, January 1989 **3–40**

Groups of 30 to 40 infants with respiratory distress syndrome received either surfactant or standard ventilatory therapy. Treatment with surfactant not only lowered mortality from 29% to 8%, but also decreased the hospital stay by nearly a week. Although average total hospital charges were similar in the 2 groups, the cost of producing a surviving infant was nearly $20,000 less when surfactant was used. The biggest savings was a decrease in ancillary charges in the first hospital week.

▶ *Several multicentered trials are now underway in which artificial surfactant is provided to premature newborn infants with respiratory distress syndrome as part of standard ventilatory therapy. Most studies have reported results similar to those presented by Maniscalco et al., documenting that surfactant lowers mortality markedly and decreases the amount of time that the newborn infant must be hospitalized. Within the next year it is quite likely that artificial surfactant will be approved by the Food and Drug Administration for use in patients who are not included in a research protocol. Although the drug will not eliminate the occurrence of hyaline membrane disease, it should diminish the morbidity and mortality related to this debilitating condition.*

ECMO: Regional Evaluation of Need and Applicability of Selection Criteria

Cole CH, Jillson E, Kessler D
Am J Dis Child 142:1320–1324, December 1988 **3–41**

The felicitous acronym for extracorporeal membrane oxygenation, ECMO, describes a method of extrathoracic cardiopulmonary bypass used to treat severe respiratory failure in neonates. A feasibility study at 2 tertiary intensive care nurseries used accepted eligibility criteria: birth weight of more than 2 kg, gestational age of more than 34 weeks, postnatal age of less than 1 week, and a need for maximal ventilatory assistance. Extensive intracranial bleeding and major coagulopathy excluded infants from ECMO. In a series of 35 potential candidates, no criterion accurately predicted survival with conventional ventilatory therapy. Selecting infants for ECMO remains a considerable problem. The best approach is to minimize severe neonatal asphyxia and improve conventional management.

▶ *The use of ECMO for the treatment of severe neonatal asphyxia is highly controversial. The technique is difficult to perform, requires the availability of highly sophisticated personnel in intensive care settings, and is not uniformly successful. The current study attempted to evaluate whether selection criteria could be derived to predict accurately the survival of patients with conventional ventilatory therapy compared with those who might require ECMO. No predictive criteria could be established. Although ECMO may be of value for selected infants in whom other forms of therapy have failed, it cannot yet be recommended as a routine treatment for neonatal asphyxia.*

Liver Transplantation in Infants and Children

Kalayoglu M, Stratta RJ, Sollinger HW, et al
J Pediatr Surg 24:70–76, January 1989 **3–42**

Fourteen infants and 11 older children received orthotopic liver transplants, usually because of biliary atresia. Seven patients had surgery on an urgent basis. The operation took about 7 hours on average. Two patients each had hepatic artery thromboses and biliary complications. Despite frequent rejection episodes only 1 graft was lost from this cause. Similarly, none of the many infectious complications led to graft loss. Both patient and graft survival rates exceed 80% at 16 months. All of the survivors have been totally rehabilitated and have normal liver function. As the results continue to improve, liver transplantation becomes the primary approach to selected patients with biliary atresia. In addition, infants in end-stage acute or chronic liver failure now can undergo transplantation at an early stage.

▶ *Biliary atresia may be characterized by lack of intrahepatic bile ducts, lack of extrahepatic bile ducts, or both. Before the advent of the Kasai surgical procedure, the disease was uniformly fatal. Even when the surgical procedure was performed, although morbidity and mortality rates varied from center to center, results were generally less than satisfactory. The recent improvement in survival rates after liver transplantation, as outlined in this article, supports the view of the authors, namely, that liver transplantation should be the primary approach to selected patients with biliary atresia. Transplantation is generally reserved for infants weighing more than 4 kg who have end-stage or chronic liver failure. Transplantation is now also indicated for children with liver failure caused by tyrosinemia, fulminant hepatic failure, Wilson's disease, and other selected inherited disorders characterized by chronic liver failure.*

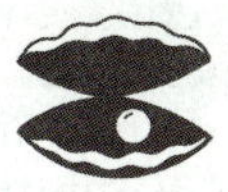

Hemolytic anemia noted in a child after a tick bite that occurred on Martha's Vineyard, Nantucket Island, or Cape Cod (Massachusetts) should suggest the possible diagnosis of babesiosis, a parasitic disease caused by *Babesia microti*.

Minor Anomalies in Offspring of Epileptic Mothers

Gaily E, Granström M-L, Hiilesmaa V, et al
J Pediatr 112:520–529, April 1988 **3–43**

At age 5 years, 120 children of epileptic mothers, most of them exposed to phenytoin, were assessed for minor physical anomalies, as were 105 control children. An excess of anomalies comprising the hydantoin syndrome was confirmed in children of epileptic mothers and in the mothers themselves. The only anomalies associated with phenytoin exposure were hypertelorism and digital hypoplasia. The other anomalies apparently are genetically linked with epilepsy. No child had major life-threatening anomalies. The risk of minor anomalies does not contraindicate either pregnancy for epileptic women or phenytoin treatment during pregnancy.

▶ *There is a reluctance to use any drug in the pregnant woman because of a fear that it will produce congenital anomalies in the newborn infant. This fear was particularly heightened during an era in which thalidomide was prescribed for many women who subsequently gave birth to infants with major limb deformities. Many children and adults have epilepsy, and it is necessary to continue anticonvulsant therapy during pregnancy. This paper is indeed welcome because it documents that phenytoin can be given for control of seizures in the pregnant woman with a risk of only minor anomalies in the newborn infant, namely, wide-set eyes and some hypoplasia of the digits. It would be ideal to find a form of anticonvulsant therapy that could be provided during pregnancy that resulted in no congenital anomalies.*

Frequency and Severity of Infections in Day Care

Wald ER, Dashefsky B, Byers C, et al
J Pediatr 112:540–546, April 1988 **3–44**

Today, nearly half of all American women with young infants work outside the home and many send their children to day care. How great is the toll of communicable illness that results? Forty-five children in day care were compared with 40 in group care and 159 in home care for 12 to 18 months. Children staying at home had fewer infectious episodes than those in day care. About 67% of the day-care group had 4 or more severe illnesses, compared with only 21% of children cared for at home. Respiratory infections were far more frequent in children cared for away from home. Also, 21% of children in day care had to be hospitalized for myringotomy and tube placement. It must be said, however, that children in day care may become immune to certain infectious agents and thus will be protected in years to come.

▶ *Families in which both parents work, or single-parent families, are becoming the norm rather than the exception. These societal trends have resulted in the widespread use of day-care centers for children of working parents. As anticipated, children in day-care centers more frequently have respiratory infections and illnesses of greater severity than those not placed in such centers. Physicians should be taught to advise parents of children who will be placed in day-care centers about the potential for infections such as* Haemophilus influenzae, *meningococcal disease, shigellosis, cryptosporidiosis, cytomegalovirus disease,* Giardia lamblia *infection, and a large number of upper respiratory viral infections. Many of these infections can be prevented by simple attention to sanitary procedures, including careful handwashing and careful cleansing of diaper changing areas within each center. Parents who seek to place a child in a day-care center should visit it to inspect the sanitary conditions, and they should assess the knowledge of the day-care center employees and director with regard to prevention of infectious diseases.*

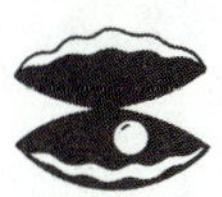

A bulging anterior fontanelle associated with cloudy corneas in a 3-month-old infant should suggest a diagnosis of cystic fibrosis. Vitamin A malabsorption may be noted in patients with cystic fibrosis and cause pseudotumor cerebri and epithelial changes in the cornea.

Human Parvovirus B19 Infection in a Day Care Worker

Noel GJ, Gary GW Jr
Pediatr Infect Dis J 7:880, December 1988 **3–45**

Children at day-care centers are at risk of contracting several infectious diseases, one of which is erythema infectiosum, the so-called fifth disease. Caretakers as well as children may acquire some of these infections. A woman aged 25 who worked at a family day-care center noted a lacy red rash on her thighs and trunk, followed in 5 days by fever, sore throat, and swollen hands and knees. Two children, 1 of them the patient's daughter, had findings of erythema infectiosum at this time and 3 others later were infected. Convalescent patient serum contained elevated titers of antibody to human parvovirus B19. If a pregnant caretaker or a person with hemolytic anemia were to contract erythema infectiosum, the outcome could be serious.

▶ *Parvoviruses as a cause of childhood infection were not documented until 4 or 5 years ago. At that time, a series of reports appeared documenting that parvoviruses can produce a disorder known as erythema infectiosum (previously classified as a disease presumably of infectious etiology) as well as aplastic anemia. This paper documents that erythema infectiosum (fifth disease) is related to human parvovirus B19. Of great import is the documentation that this disease may produce epidemic infection in day-care centers. Health care workers should also know that pregnant women and patients with hemolytic anemia may be at increased risk for serious problems after parvovirus infection.* *(For more on parvovirus, see Abstract 3–28.)*

Epidemiology of Human Bites to Children in a Day-Care Center

Garrard J, Leland N, Smith DK
Am J Dis Child 142:643–650, June 1988 **3–46**

Would you enroll a child in day care if you knew that there is nearly a 50–50 chance that he or she will be bitten by another child? A review was made of bite injuries in 224 infants, toddlers, and preschoolers at a day-care center. More than 100 children received nearly 350 bites. Toddlers were bitten most often and preschoolers least often. Among the toddlers, boys received more bite injuries than girls. Children enrolled the longest at the center were the most likely to be injured. Apparently, the upper extremity was most appealing to biters of all ages. No child was taken to a physician or an emergency room.

▶ *Infections in day-care centers have received a great deal of attention. This is one of the few articles to describe and study the issue of human bites to children in day-care centers. The results are astounding in that there was a 50% chance that any child enrolled in a day-care center would be the victim of a human bite. Infection after a human bite can be quite serious and prompt medical attention is important. Many specialists believe that after the wound has been thoroughly cleansed, treatment with Augmentin (a combination of ampicillin and β-lactamase inhibitor) or Timentin for 5 days may be useful in preventing secondary infection.*

Management of Illness and Temporary Disability in Children Enrolled in Day-Care Centers: The Health House Experience

Chang A, Zeledon-Friendly A, Britt A, et al
Am J Dis Child 142:651–655, June 1988 **3–47**

When children at day-care centers become ill or temporarily disabled, alternate arrangements for care are needed. In some states ill children must be removed from the center. A Health House was established by the Pomona, California school district adjacent to a day-care center. During a single school year, about 100 children were treated under the program for disorders similar to those seen in the physician's office. The average daily salary savings for the working parent was $40. Apart from this practical aspect, guilt feelings are lessened for parents who know that their children are being well cared for. Another approach would be to liberalize parental leave during a child's illness.

▸ *The problem of what to do with the child who becomes ill while attending a day-care center has assumed national significance. Parents either have to remain home, with an associated loss of income, or find another caretaker, or, occasionally, bring the child to the day-care center despite the illness. It is this latter action that is responsible for much of the spread of infection in day-care centers. In recent years a relatively modest number of centers have been developed to care for children who become ill away from home. The availability of these centers should help to diminish the incidence of infectious diseases in the normal day-care center; however, the likelihood that a child with diarrheal illness who might infect a patient with respiratory illness in one of these alternative day-care center facilities has never been studied and is an important consideration. Another approach to the problem has been the development of centers for sick children in a wing of a hospital that has unoccupied beds. This latter arrangement provides significant comfort for parents in that they know that their child will be cared for by experienced personnel.*

Milk Production by Mothers of Premature Infants

Hopkinson JM, Schanler RJ, Garza C
Pediatrics 81:815–820, June 1988 **3–48**

It seems best for an infant of very low birth weight to receive milk from its own mother early on. The problem is that to accelerate growth in these infants a lot of milk is needed. Patterns of lactation were studied in mothers of healthy infants to find the optimal milk production. Milk volume was highest when milk expression began shortly after delivery. With at least 5 expressions each day and pumping for a total of 100 minutes or more, milk production was optimal. As always, there is individual variation; some women need more than 15 minutes to empty each breast.

▶ *It is well documented that maternal milk is the best source of food for the very-low-birth-weight infant. Lack of information suggested that very-low-birth-weight infants might have immature enzymes in the gastrointestinal tract that could impair absorption of maternal milk. More recent data suggest that this is not the case except under unusual circumstances in infants of 24 to 30 weeks' gestation. There has been a proliferation of milk banks to store maternal milk for feeding to the newborn infant who remains in a neonatal intensive care unit for an extensive period of time, and this practice will undoubtedly increase.*

Birth Weight and Childhood Growth

Binkin NJ, Yip R, Fleshood L, et al
Pediatrics 82:828–834, December 1988 **3–49**

Infants of low birth weight do grow rapidly, but they fail to achieve the same size as their normal-sized peers. A review of birth records for a 10-year period in Tennessee confirmed that smaller infants were likely to remain lighter and shorter throughout childhood. This was especially true of infants whose growth was retarded in utero. Larger infants, on the other hand, were more likely to become obese. Birth weight proves to be a strong predictor of weight and height in early childhood for all children, not just those of low birth weight. Intrauterine growth retardation is more closely linked with short stature and underweight than is prematurity.

▶ *Standard textbooks teach that premature infants exhibit "catch-up" growth and are not necessarily shorter in size or lower in weight than infants who are born at term with "normal" body weights. The current study by Binkin and associates suggests that these previous concepts are inaccurate. Birth weight proved to be a strong predictor of weight and height in early childhood for all children, not just those of low birth weight. Even though infants of low birth weight grew rapidly and had some "catch-up" growth, they failed to reach the same size as their normal-sized peers. Although parents of low-birth-weight children can be informed about the possibility of "catch-up" growth, they should no longer be told that their children will achieve the same height and weight of other siblings in the same family who are born at term.*

Growth Hormone Assessment and Short-Term Treatment With Growth Hormone in Turner Syndrome

Lin T-H, Kirkland JL, Kirkland RT
J Pediatr 112:919–922, June 1988 **3–50**

Patients with Turner's syndrome have abnormal growth as children and are short in adulthood. The cause is uncertain, but disordered growth hormone (GH) secretion may be responsible. Ten prepubertal children with Turner's syndrome had a mean GH concentration similar to that of control children. During treatment with Somatrem, 0.1 mg/kg 3 times weekly, growth velocity increased from 2.9 to 6.5 cm per year. The growth response was not predicted by the mean 24-hour GH level at baseline or by GH responses to clonidine and glucagon.

► *This is the first study documenting that children with Turner's syndrome can be helped by the use of synthetic GH. Improvement in the height of children with short stature, regardless of its etiology, is most important. Many studies have documented that children who are unusually short suffer from the emotional consequences of their disease, particularly during elementary and junior high school years. Sociologic studies have documented that the earning potential of individuals who are more than 2 SD below the mean in height is far less than those who are close to or above the mean adult height in selected population groups. It is graftifying to know that children with Turner's syndrome can be helped by therapy with human GH, so that one of the many difficulties that they may ultimately encounter as a result of their complex genetic disorder may be eliminated.*

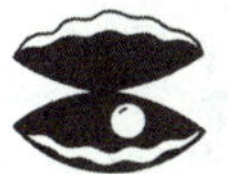

Enlarged corneas (>11 mm in diameter) in a newborn infant who is incessantly irritable should suggest a diagnosis of congenital glaucoma.

Long-term Auxologic Effect of Human Growth Hormone

Bundak R, Hindmarsh PC, Smith PJ, et al
J Pediatr 112:875–879, June 1988 **3–51**

Intuitively, when growth hormone (GH) is begun at an earlier age it would seem that better long-term growth results. The "auxologic" (from the Greek *auxe,* to increase) effects of GH were studied in 58 prepubertal and 20 pubertal children with idiopathic hormone deficiency. Subcutaneous doses of 2 to 10 units were given 2 to 7 times a week for up to 5 years. In the prepubertal children, height velocity increased most in the first year of treatment, but it was always significantly greater than in the year before treatment. The height deficit at the end of treatment was greater in patients who were pubertal at the time treatment began. It obviously is important to diagnose GH deficiency early. Treatment can prevent continuing loss of stature, but it cannot make up an existing deficit.

▶ *The advent of synthetic GH has led to a proliferation of studies designed to assess its use in many groups of children with various forms of short stature who previously would not have been considered candidates for therapy. Naturally occurring GH has always been used predominantly in children with idiopathic GH deficiency. Even these children, however, can now be treated with greater safety and less expense with synthetic GH. Bundak et al. showed that early application of naturally occurring GH is important, because it does stimulate growth; however, growth deficits cannot be made up over time if treatment is begun after puberty has started. It seems likely that the principle established in this study will foster the use of synthetic GH in these children relatively early in life.*

Cardiovascular Disease Risk Reduction for Tenth Graders: A Multiple-Factor School-Based Approach

Killen JD, Telch MJ, Robinson TN, et al
JAMA 260:1728–1733, Sept 23/30, 1988 **3–52**

If one risk behavior—smoking—can be reduced in high school students, why not multiple risk factors? Almost 1,500 10th-graders at 4 California high schools had 20 classroom sessions discussing smoking, nutrition, physical activity, stress, and how to solve personal problems. Each module provided information on health practices and taught the cognitive and behavioral skills that make it possible to alter personal behaviors. The children practiced specific skills to improve their performance. Intervention led to more exercise and a more judicious choice of snacks. In addition, fewer students returned to regular smoking. There were positive effects of intervention on heart rate, body mass index, and skinfold thicknesses. School-based primary prevention education is definitely worthwhile.

▶ *The current article is one of a very few that assess the effectiveness of early intervention in the form of health education to deal with the factors that are most likely to contribute to heart disease in adult life. The effect of an educational program on heart rate, body mass index, and skinfold thickness were positive. Children were led to choose snacks more judiciously and exercise more frequently. It is far less costly to prevent hypertension and heart disease than to treat it; also, some of the frequently used high-cost procedures such as coronary bypass surgery may not be as effective as previously believed. All physicians should encourage preventive health practices throughout life as the most cost-effective approach to medical care.*

Factors Affecting the Relationship Between Childhood and Adult Cholesterol Levels: The Muscatine Study

Lauer RM, Lee J, Clarke WR
Pediatrics 82:309–318, September 1988 **3–53**

Most other studies tracking cholesterol levels through young adulthood have not used the same population throughout. In this series of 2,500 individuals, cholesterol levels were compared at ages 8–18 and 20–30 years. Elevated cholesterol levels in childhood were in fact associated with high adult values. The risk began to increase when childhood levels were above the 50th percentile. When they were at the 90th percentile, at least 25% of young adults had high cholesterol levels. Adverse cholesterol and lipoprotein values also were more likely when a person became obese, smoked cigarettes, or used oral contraception. If children with high cholesterol levels know that they are at special risk of coronary heart disease, they may agree to do whatever is necessary to lower that risk.

▶ *This is the first study to track cholesterol levels in the same group of individuals from young childhood into early adult life. Previous studies did not use the same population groups to assess normal cholesterol levels in individuals of different ages. This study clearly documents that children who have a high cholesterol level at the age of 8 years are far more likely to have a similarly elevated cholesterol level at ages 20–30 years. This study provides an important stimulus to screen all children for cholesterol, total lipids, and high- and low-density lipoprotein levels, and to prescribe appropriate dietary therapy for those whose cholesterol levels fall more than 1 SD above the mean early in life. Explanation to the child and his parents of the increased risk of maintaining an elevated cholesterol level can be used to reinforce the advice to follow a heart-healthy diet throughout life.*

Child Molestation and Pedophilia: An Overview for the Physician

Fuller AK
JAMA 261:602–606, Jan 27, 1989 **3–54**

More than 100,000 children in the United States, and perhaps as many as half a million, are sexually molested each year. Symptoms may appear some time after the event, and the victim's life can be pervasively damaged. Contrary to what is often thought, pedophiles typically impose their wishes in many different forms on their victims. The first diagnostic measure is to distinguish between primary pedophilia and some psychiatric disorder having child molestation as a secondary feature. Drugs, psychotherapy, and behavioral therapy are available, but obviously the key is primary prevention. Youngsters, the general public, and the medical community all need to learn how to identify abused children and how to detect potential molesters before they commit an offense.

▶ *Sexual molestation is one of many forms of child abuse that appear to be increasing in frequency in the United States. The diagnosis is often difficult to establish because (1) the child may be too young to report what has transpired; (2) the child may be too fearful to report the event; or (3) the psychological symptoms that the child may display months or years later may not be related temporally by child, parents, or physician to the previous event. All physicians must remember that reporting actual or suspected abuse to child protection authorities is a statutory requirement, not a substitute for referring both the victim and the abuser for psychiatric or psychological assessment and therapy.*

4

Psychiatry

Prevalence of Mental Illness

One-Month Prevalence of Mental Disorders in the United States: Based on Five Epidemiologic Catchment Area Sites

Regier DA, Boyd JH, Burke JD Jr, et al
Arch Gen Psychiatry 45:977–986, November 1988 **4–1**

One-month prevalence rates of mental disorder were determined in community samples totaling more than 18,500 persons at 5 sites in the NIMH Epidemiologic Catchment Area program. Fifteen percent of the population aged 18 and older had at least 1 mental disorder (Table 1). Most disorders other than those of cognition were more common in persons younger than age 45. Substance abuse and antisocial personality were more prevalent in men and disorders of affect and somatization in women. If similar studies are done in international and cross-cultural settings, the contributions of biologic, psychological, and cultural differences to various mental disorders will be clarified.

▶ *There are 2 striking findings in this report of the best epidemiologic study yet done on the prevalence of mental disorders among Americans. First is the high percentage (15%) of Americans who have diagnosable mental illnesses at any one time and, second, is the high number of these who have phobic (6%) or affective (5%) disorders. Over a lifetime, however, substance abuse disorders rise to the top (16%).*

The Prevalence of Bulimia Nervosa in the US College Student Population

Drewnowski A, Hopkins SA, Kessler RC
Am J Public Health 78:1322–1325, October 1988 **4–2**

A phone survey of 1,000 students at 53 colleges and universities showed that 1% of women and 0.2% of men were bulimic. Bulimia was most prevalent, at a rate of 2.2%, in undergraduate women living in group housing on campus. The bulimic

TABLE 1.

Comparison of Standardized 1-Month, 6-Month, and Lifetime Prevalence Rates of DIS/*DSM-III* Disorders per 100 Persons Aged 18 Years and Older

Disorders	Rate, % (SE) 1 mo	6 mo	Lifetime
Any DIS disorder covered	15.4 (0.4)	19.1 (0.4)	32.2 (0.5)
Any DIS disorder except cognitive impairment, substance use disorder, and antisocial personality	11.2 (0.3)	13.1 (0.4)	19.6 (0.4)
Any DIS disorder except phobia	11.2 (0.3)	14.0 (0.4)	25.2 (0.5)
Any DIS disorder except substance use disorders	12.6 (0.3)	14.8 (0.4)	22.1 (0.4)
Any DIS disorder except substance use or phobia	8.3 (0.3)	9.4 (0.3)	13.8 (0.4)
Substance use disorders	3.8 (0.2)	6.0 (0.3)	16.4 (0.4)
Alcohol abuse/dependence	2.8 (0.2)	4.7 (0.2)	13.3 (0.4)
Drug abuse/dependence	1.3 (0.1)	2.0 (0.1)	5.9 (0.2)
Schizophrenic/schizophreniform disorders	0.7 (0.1)	0.9 (0.1)	1.5 (0.1)
Schizophrenia	0.6 (0.1)	0.8 (0.1)	1.3 (0.1)
Schizophreniform disorder	0.1 (0.0)	0.1 (0.0)	0.1 (0.0)
Affective disorders	5.1 (0.2)	5.8 (0.3)	8.3 (0.3)
Manic episode	0.4 (0.1)	0.5 (0.1)	0.8 (0.1)
Major depressive episode	2.2 (0.2)	3.0 (0.2)	5.8 (0.3)
Dysthymia†	3.3 (0.2)	3.3 (0.2)	3.3 (0.2)
Anxiety disorders	7.3 (0.3)	8.9 (0.3)	14.6 (0.4)
Phobia	6.2 (0.2)	7.7 (0.3)	12.5 (0.3)
Panic	0.5 (0.1)	0.8 (0.1)	1.6 (0.1)
Obsessive-compulsive	1.3 (0.1)	1.5 (0.1)	2.5 (0.2)
Somatization disorder	0.1 (0.0)	0.1 (0.0)	0.1 (0.0)
Personality disorder, antisocial personality	0.5 (0.1)	0.8 (0.1)	2.5 (0.2)
Cognitive impairment (severe)†	1.3 (0.1)	1.3 (0.1)	1.3 (0.1)

Rates for all sites are standardized to the age, sex, and race distribution of the 1980 noninstitutionalized population of the United States aged 18 years and older. *DIS,* Diagnostic Interview Schedule; *DSM-III, Diagnostic and Statistical Manual of Mental Disorders,* ed III.

*Dysthymia and cognitive impairment have no recency information; therefore, the rates are the same for all 3 time periods.

(Courtesy of Regier DA, Boyd JH, Burke JD Jr, et al: *Arch Gen Psychiatry* 45:977–986, November 1988.)

women were heavier than the population mean and wished to be thinner than the group ideal. Bulimic behaviors such as binge eating were somewhat more frequent than a DSM-III-R diagnosis of bulimia nervosa. Only 2 of the 5 bulimics interviewed have sought professional help. This may explain in part why high prevalence figures are not matched by a high number of treatment referrals.

▶ *In the 1989 edition of* Roundsmanship *(p 139) I commented on a study showing that 40% of college women engaged in binge eating, but only 1% could be diagnosed as bulimic by* DSM-III, *illustrating the difference between symptoms and diseases. The present article not only confirms the rate (1%), but reveals another commonplace in psychiatry: the gap between those whose disease is diagnosed and those seeking treatment (40%).*

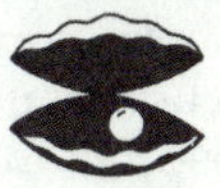

All pain is an intrapsychic state.

Psychiatric Diagnoses in Patients Who Have Chronic Fatigue Syndrome

Kruesi MJP, Dale J, Straus SE
J Clin Psychiatry 50:53–56, February 1989 **4–3**

A role for Epstein-Barr virus infection in chronic fatigue syndrome remains unproved. Could the disorder, which comprises debilitating fatigability, depression, and difficulty in concentrating as well as low-grade fever, sore throat, musculoskeletal pains, and headache, be psychiatric in nature? Twenty-eight patients meeting CDC criteria for chronic fatigue syndrome did indeed have increased rates of psychiatric illness, which more often preceded than followed the chronic fatigue. Depressive episodes and simple phobia were most frequent.

▶ *Oh boy! The authors tilt toward the conclusion that the high lifetime prevalence of psychiatric disorders, 75% in chronic fatigue patients (as revealed in Abstract 4–1) as opposed to only 32% in the general public, and their antecedent occurrence, suggest their role in the pathogenesis of this puzzling disease. Be careful how you quote this, though; the authors are careful to stress that studies mainly support the role of infectious diseases in delaying recovery,* not *in causing illness.*

Psychosocial Variables and Hypertension: A New Look at an Old Controversy

Sommers-Flanagan J, Greenberg RP
J Nerv Ment Dis 177:15–24, January 1989 **4–4**

From more than 100 research reports appearing in the past 6 years, as well as numerous texts and reviews, it is clear that hypertensive patients have problems in identifying and expressing aggressive feelings. They also tend to be anxious and isolated, and to have strong physiologic reactions to interpersonal situations, especially when communication is necessary. Hypertensives often use denial and repression to cope with their conflicts. Because there obviously is a psychosocial side to hypertension, it is logical to consider psychosocial interventions. Some possibilities: Provide social skills training; teach stress management and communication skills; offer insight through psychotherapy.

▶ *When I was a medical student, hypertension was presented as a "classical psychosomatic disease." More recently, its medical pathogenesis has chased this belief into disrepute. Now, however, after reviewing the voluminous literature on the disease (from 1979 to 1986), the authors suggest that we respect the convincing research findings and intervene psychosocially as well as pharmacologically. Makes sense to me.*

Insulin Misuse: A Review of an Overlooked Psychiatric Problem

Kaminer Y, Robbins DR
Psychosomatics 30:19–24, Winter 1989 **4–5**

Suicides may well be more frequent in diabetics because the diagnosis embraces the prominent risk factors of adolescence/young adulthood and physical illness itself. Apart from the diabetic patient using insulin suicidally, relatives may occasionally do so. Variations on this theme: insulin misuse leading to factitious hypoglycemia; child maltreatment by injecting insulin; and insulin as a substance of abuse.

▶ *Most of us are all too aware of the potential misuses of certain medications (e.g., narcotics and sleeping pills) by our patients, but we may miss abuse involving a substance such as insulin, prescribed to remedy so clear-cut a medical condition. The fact that there is such a high rate of recurrence is all the more reason to be on the alert.*

Physicians' Emotional Reactions to Patients

Smith RC, Zimny GH
Psychosomatics 29:392–397, Fall 1988 **4–6**

What is it in patients that experienced internists react to most strongly? A sample of 60 physicians indicated that perceived threats to their integrity or self-esteem incited the strongest emotional reaction. Next was the demanding or upset patient, or one making undue demands on the physician. Circumstances that could not be altered, or that did not relate directly to the physician, proved to be relatively neutral. If, as educators believe, the physician-patient relationship is indeed important, doctors' emotional responses should be addressed during training.

▶ *This study is flawed scientifically by an unacceptably low response rate (20%) and the lack of information concerning to what degree physicians actually acted on their feelings. However, it serves as a useful reminder that physicians, although like everyone else in not enjoying criticism, must not act like everyone else on such feelings lest they endanger their relationship with the patient and his or her treatment.*

The Physician's Responsibility Toward Hopelessly Ill Patients: A Second Look

Wanzer SH, Federman DD, Adelstein SJ, et al
N Engl J Med 320:844–849, March 30, 1989 **4–7**

Some formerly controversial practices such as "do not resuscitate" orders now are commonplace, and the courts are approaching the view that patients are entitled to be allowed to die, even if they are not in pain or terminally ill. Dying at home is private and dignified, and makes things easier for both the patient and the bereaved. Flexible, continuously adjusted care is the key to controlling pain, fear, and anxiety. As death moves closer, measures to minimize pain should be intensified. Before helping a patient commit suicide the physician must be certain that there is no recourse and that treatable depression is not present. The public response when asked about euthanasia is increasingly favorable.

▶ *This paper was written after its 12 authors spent 3 days discussing a variety of ticklish, if not taboo, issues about hopelessly ill patients. The teaching point here is that all issues concerning the terminally ill, from pain relief to euthanasia, deserve a great deal of thought and debate whenever they come up, especially as public and professional opinion keeps shifting.*

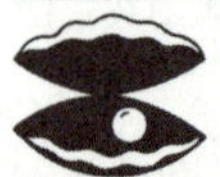

Hypnosis was originally explained as "animal magnetism" affecting the subject and hypnotist.

The Suicidal, Terminally Ill Patient With Depression

Leibenluft E, Goldberg RL
Psychosomatics 29:379–386, Fall 1988 **4–8**

Six terminally ill patients who were suicidal were looked at closely in the hope of finding some coherent approach. Four patients attempted suicide when psychological and physical discomfort was mounting because of progressive illness or its treatment. Four patients overdosed with analgesics or psychotropic drugs. Both cognitive and vegetative symptoms were prevalent in these patients. All but 1 of the patients had a good to excellent response after an average stay of 3 weeks in a psychiatric unit. In several instances the family played a critical role in treatment. Rather than viewing suicidal behavior as an inevitable sequel to serious physical illness, it should be managed as it would be in physically healthy persons.

▶ *Too frequently, we assume that suicidal feelings or actions in the terminally ill are absolutely rational. This paper reminds us not to impose our reasoning on the patient—he or she may be depressed and respond well to antidepressants. On the other hand, we should also go farther than medicating. Giving the patient control over some parts of his or her life may be crucial.*

Pitfalls and Pratfalls in Consultation-Liaison Psychiatry in a General Hospital

Rowe CJ, Billings RF, Pohlman ER, et al
Can J Psychiatry 33:294–298, May 1988 **4–9**

Only recently has in-hospital psychiatric consultation become a matter of course. All agree that an "integrative" approach is important, but the fact remains that medical staff and psychiatrists often have strong reservations about each other's role in managing patients. A generally worded consultation request may include a hidden agenda, and it is up to the consultant to find out what is really being sought. It is most helpful to get input from the nursing staff before seeing the patient, as well as to review all available records. If the patient can view the psychiatrist as a member of the medical team, acceptance of the consultation will come easier. Educational initiatives should be undertaken in a spirit of collaboration, not as dogmatic or competitive teaching. Special care is needed if there are medicolegal aspects to a consultation.

▶ *How often do we turn to a consultant when we're fed up with a patient rather than simply baffled? This calls not so much for diagnostic acumen with the patient as for detective work, often involving the staff. As overworked as we are on clinical rotations, looking closely at our reasoning behind the consultation may be the most effective and efficient way of solving the problem.*

AIDS and HIV Infection

HIV Infection Associated With Symptoms Indistinguishable From Functional Psychosis

Buhrich N, Cooper DA, Freed E
Br J Psychiatry 152:649–653, 1988 **4–10**

The occasional patient with HIV infection has signs of functional psychosis, but impaired cognition soon is evident. An AIDS patient and 2 others with AIDS-related complex were seen who had psychotic symptoms but normal cognition. Two patients had schizophreniform psychosis and 1 had a manic episode. Because HIV is neuropathic and can produce organic brain disorders, it is likely that neuropathic effects explain the functional psychosis in these patients.

▶ *At the June 1989 International Conference on AIDS in Montreal, evidence was presented that it was highly unusual for AIDS patients to present first with neurologic/psychiatric symptoms—a finding that is reassuring to those concerned about travel safety and so on. However, as this study shows, patients can present with a functional psychosis in addition to the usual cognitive impairment.*

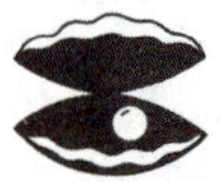

Sleepwalking and night terrors occur during non-rapid eye movement sleep and are not a result of dreaming.

Consultation-Liaison Psychiatry and HIV-Related Disorders

Fernandez F, Holmes VF, Levy JK, et al
Hosp Community Psychiatry 40:146–153, February 1989 **4–11**

Many AIDS patients have a wide range of psychosocial and neuropsychiatric complications (Table 2). One implication for the consultation-liaison psychiatrist is that any psychiatric symptoms in a patient who may have HIV infection must be considered to be organic until proved otherwise. Social abandonment is a special fear of these patients; they frequently feel guilty, despondent, and demoralized. Psychostimulants are recommended for depressed, cognitively impaired patients. The concerned psychiatrist can take measures to prevent staff burnout, always a possibility when dealing with AIDS patients.

▶ *In line with the comment accompanying Abstract 4–10, these authors demonstrate the wide variety of symptoms an AIDS patient may display at various stages of the illness (Table 2). The point this paper brings home most strongly, however, is how many issues we must consider (psychiatric, diagnostic, social, ethical, and legal) when assessing and treating persons with AIDS.*

TABLE 2.
Early and Late Manifestations of the AIDS Dementia Complex

Early manifestations
- Complaints, symptoms
  - Memory loss
  - Impaired concentration
  - Comprehension difficulties
  - Conceptual confusion
  - Apathy
  - Depressive mood
  - Agitation
  - Psychotic features
  - Unsteady gait
  - Tremor
  - Clumsiness
  - Motor weakness
- Signs, findings
  - Psychomotor slowing
  - Memory dysfunction
  - Impairment of information processing
  - Mild to moderate constructional difficulties
  - Visuospatial disorganization
  - Mild frontal lobe dysfunction
  - Dysgraphia
  - Dysarthria, dysnomia
  - Mild or moderate cerebellar dysfunction
  - Hyperreflexia

Late manifestations
- Global cognitive dysfunction
- Mutism
- Aphasia
- Amnestic features
- Frontal lobe disturbance
- Dominant and nondominant parietal lobe signs
- Organic hallucinosis
- Weakness
- Spasticity
- Dyskinesia
- Parkinsonism
- Ataxia
- Myoclonus
- Incontinence
- Seizures

(Adapted from Navia BA, Jordan BD, Price RW: *Ann Neurol* 19:517–524, 1986. Courtesy of Fernandez F, Holmes VF, Levy JK, et al: *Hosp Community Psychiatry* 40:146–153, February 1989.)

Counseling for HIV Testing

Perry SW, Markowitz JC
Hosp Community Psychiatry 39:731–739, July 1988 **4–12**

The many persons who seek HIV testing would be well served if a coherent strategy for counseling were available. At the outset, the meaning of the test is explained and the limits of confidentiality discussed. The client must know that the mutual decision to test can be made only after the risks and benefits are carefully considered. Coping capacity and available support are best assessed before test results are made known. In post-test counseling, attempts are made to reduce distress if necessary. Clients are told about how to prevent infection, and any further questions are answered. A silent person may actually be numb or embarrassed; inquiring into follow-up care provides an opening for a discussion of immediate plans or self-destructive impulses.

▶ *People talk about HIV counseling as if it's like the college selection process—predictable, static, relatively uncomplicated, and requiring minimal skills or training. It's not. The authors spend 30 to 90 minutes before the test and 2 hours or more afterward explaining the results. They cover a gamut of topics, concerns, and fears. And, they are very sophisticated. Many patients want their doctors involved, so be prepared.*

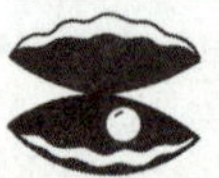

Some AIDS patients have depression as their initial complaint.

Response of HIV-Related Depression to Psychostimulants: Case Reports

Fernandez F, Levy JK, Galizzi H
Hosp Community Psychiatry 39:628–631, June 1988 **4–13**

Patients infected with HIV who are depressed frequently improve when aggressively treated with stimulants, even if cognition is impaired. Four representative patients responded positively to methylphenidate and dextroamphetamine, starting on the first day of treatment. Cognitive and behavioral problems also lessened with stimulant treatment, and none of the usual adverse effects occurred. Existing dyskinesia, however, did become worse when dextroamphetamine was given. Stimulant therapy can help these patients participate in rehabilitative activities and renew disrupted personal relationships.

▶ *This paper brings home the old but oft-forgotten point that persons who are depressed respond well to psychostimulants, such as amphetamines. In fact, some psychiatrists use these drugs to predict responsiveness to antidepressants. It should be no surprise, then, that persons with AIDS-related depression also respond. Despite the small "n," these were promising results.*

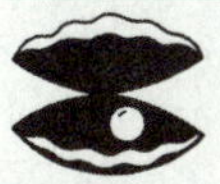

Amphetamines for treating hyperactivity have been used since the 1930s.

Stress Disorders

Health Status of Vietnam Veterans: I. Psychosocial Characteristics

Centers for Disease Control Vietnam Experience Study
JAMA 259:2701–2707, May 13, 1988 **4–14**

Many Vietnam veterans are concerned that their experiences may have compromised their health and possibly that of their children. A multidimensional study queried groups of 7,000 to 8,000 Vietnam and non-Vietnam veterans similar in education, income, and marital status. Depression, anxiety, and alcohol abuse or dependence were more prevalent in the Vietnam veterans. About 15% of this group had combat-related posttraumatic stress disorder at some time. Neither personal characteristics nor current physical health can explain the especially high prevalence of psychological disorders in Vietnam veterans. Their social and economic attainments are not lower as a result, but it should be recognized that, even in the overall context of combat, the Vietnam experience was particularly trying.

▶ *This Centers for Disease Control study hammers home again the devastating impact of the Vietnam War on a large number of individuals who served there. The teaching point of this study, however, is that there is no one resultant symptom or disease (e.g., posttraumatic stress disorder); there are several. Taking a military history is crucial in men 35 to 50 years old.*

Diagnostic and Psychopharmacological Treatment Characteristics of 536 Inpatients With Posttraumatic Stress Disorder

Faustman WO, White PA
J Nerv Ment Dis 177:154–159, March 1989 **4–15**

This large series of male veterans with a DSM-III diagnosis of posttraumatic stress disorder (PTSD) had, as expected, high rates of alcohol and substance abuse and depression. More than half had previously been psychiatric inpatients. Nearly a third of the patients received an axis II diagnosis; borderline features were most prevalent. Half of the patients received drugs in addition to psychotherapy, usually antidepressants, neuroleptics, or β-blockers. Effective treatment of PTSD requires an understanding of the specific problems these patients experience.

▸ *Following the points made in Abstract 4–14, this study demonstrates the extent of comorbidity among Vietnam veterans in a VA Hospital. These included axis I (alcohol and drug abuse and depression) and axis II (a third had borderline personality disorder). As one might expect from such a coexistence of illnesses, treatments were also complicated.*

Posttraumatic Stress Disorder as a Consequence of the POW Experience

Speed N, Engdahl B, Schwartz J, et al
J Nerv Ment Dis 177:147–153, March 1989 **4–16**

We continue to try to learn whether premorbid personality or trauma itself contributes most to posttraumatic stress disorder (PTSD). Of 60 men who had been prisoners of war in World War II, half received a diagnosis of PTSD within a year of being repatriated; after 40 years a third of them still met criteria for the disorder. Neither preexisting psychopathology nor a family history of mental illness strongly predicted persisting PTSD.

On the other hand, being tortured and losing a lot of body weight were strong predictors.

▶ *Just as previous studies of Vietnam veterans have demonstrated that combat exposure increases the probability of PTSD developing, so does this study show that torture predicts "persisting PTSD" among World War II prisoners of war. Clearly, there is stress and there is megastress.*

Influences of Time, Ethnicity, and Attachment on Depression in Southeast Asian Refugees

Beiser M
Am J Psychiatry 145:46–51, January 1988 **4–17**

In a world with 10 million refugees, countries of asylum such as the United States and Canada must consider how to provide for the needs of displaced persons. The longer Southeast Asian refugees remain in Canada the better is their mental health. It is those who are unmarried or otherwise unattached, such as the non-Chinese refugees, who tend to be depressed a year after arriving. What's more, they continue to be depressed when social services are not provided. It is not necessary to resolve the eternal nature-nurture controversy to acknowledge the importance of the ethnic community and the supportive value of self-help groups.

▶ *There is good evidence that it is the second-generation immigrant who suffers most from cultural dislocation. But the new immigrant suffers, too, even though such difficulties erode over time. A telling point here is how much more depressed are persons who are single or unattached. This follows what we also know about the increased rate of depression and suicide in single, divorced, or widowed individuals.*

Social Relationships and Health

House JS, Landis KR, Umberson D
Science 241:540–545, July 29, 1988 **4–18**

Prospective studies controlling for health status have consistently indicated an increased mortality risk for those with inadequate social relationships. Both the quantity and quality of such relationships predict mortality for men and women in differing populations. Social isolation appears to be an important risk factor for death from widely varying causes. Current social support theories fail to provide a broad picture of the biopsychosocial mechanisms linking social relationships with health. It is evident, however, that biology and personality must affect both health and relationships. The extent and quality of social relationships also depend on broader social forces.

▶ *This report extends what we saw above (Abstract 4–17). Here, we learn 2 additional things: First, that social isolation leads to ill health in general, not just depression, and, second, that the quality of the relationship counts. To the medical student, who has a higher than average possibility of a more independent social and professional life: Beware.*

The Ravelled Sleeve of Care: Managing the Stresses of Residency Training

Colford JM Jr, McPhee SJ
JAMA 261:889–893, Feb 10, 1989 **4–19**

Residency training today is in a critical state: The lay press, house staff, and legislators all are proposing changes. Sleep deprivation probably is the greatest source of stress. Then there are "role strain" stresses related to residents' perceptions about their work and, certainly not least, the manifold stresses

TABLE 3.
The Toll of Residency Stress

Addictive Behaviors
Alcohol abuse
Drug abuse
Relationship Distress
Divorce
Broken relationships
Psychopathologic Behavior
Anxiety
Depression
Suicide
Professional Dysfunction
Job dissatisfaction
Leaves of absence
Errors
Inappropriate underconfidence or overconfidence
Cynicism
Loss of compassion

(Courtesy of Colford JM Jr, McPhee SF: *JAMA* 261:889–893, Feb 10, 1989.)

TABLE 4.
Strategies to Reduce Residency Stress

By Hospitals
To ensure adequate ancillary help
Paraprofessional support (phlebotomists, electrocardiogram technicians, etc)
Administrative support (ward clerks, messenger services, etc)
To ensure adequate benefits
Increased salaries
Expanded fringe benefits (medical, health, and disability insurance)
Other services (financial, legal, and tax counseling; child care; housing subsidies)
By Departments
Structural
"Short-stay" admissions
Physician-extenders
Grievance procedures
Educational
Increased faculty availability
Part-time positions
Formal career counseling
"Protected time"
Management counseling
By Residency Programs
Structural
"Night floats"
Reduced call frequency
Redistribute primary patient care during residency
Eliminate clinic responsibilities after nights on call
Establish backup coverage for sick residents
Educational
Training in teaching and leadership skills
Periodic performance feedback
Training in stress reduction methods
Morale
Support groups for residents and spouses
Retreats
Thorough orientation for interns
Regular social events (eg, journal clubs)
Alumni reunions with current residents

(Courtesy of Colford JM Jr, McPhee SJ: *JAMA* 261:889–893, Feb 10, 1989.)

incurred by all young professionals and by older physicians in practice. The toll of these stresses sounds loudly (Table 3), but a wide range of strategies is available for countering them (Table 4). A humanistic concern over the many deleterious effects of the stresses encountered by residents may inspire all concerned to find ways of resolving the problem.

▶ *While we're discussing the physician's life stresses and occupational hazards (see Abstract 4–18), let's look at residency. This is where stress was invented. Unfortunately, the authors' "strategies to reduce residency stress" are almost all expensive (e.g., ancillary help, administrative support, adequate benefits, reduced call, and so on), with the exception of a few (e.g., alumni reunions with current residents). Not too hopeful.*

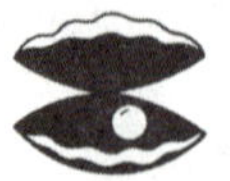

Epileptic activity, especially of the temporal lobe, can present as depression, psychosis, or personality change.

Impact of Sexual and Physical Abuse on Women's Mental Health

Mullen PE, Romans-Clarkson SE, Walton VA, et al
Lancet 1:841–845, Apr 16, 1988 **4–20**

That sexual and physical abuse of women is a major issue is a given, but what exactly are the long-term psychiatric implications? When psychiatric symptomatology was assessed in a random community sample of 2,000 women in New Zealand, a history of abuse related significantly to elevated test scores and to the number of psychiatric cases. A fifth of the women who were sexually abused as children had symptoms and these were mainly depressive. Women who were physically or sexually abused as adults also were more likely to have psychiatric disorders. The experience of abuse may be part of the reason why women are overrepresented among patients with depressive and anxiety disorders.

▶ *This is intriguing. We've known for some time that more women than men experienced certain psychiatric illnesses—specifically, depressive and anxiety disorders. We also know that many more psychiatric patients have sustained child abuse than was previously ascertained by routine history. But this is the first paper to suggest their linkage. Once again, careful histories are critical.*

Neuropsychiatric, Psychoeducational, and Family Characteristics of 14 Juveniles Condemned to Death in the United States

Lewis DO, Pincus JH, Bard B, et al
Am J Psychiatry 145:584–589, May 1988 **4–21**

What are adolescents like who commit capital crimes? Fourteen such boys sentenced to death before age 18 years were evaluated. All but 2 had been brutally abused physically, and 5 had been sodomized by older relatives. Alcoholism, drug abuse, and psychiatric hospitalization all were prevalent. Nine boys had major neurologic impairment. Seven had psychotic disorders, and 7 exhibited significant organic dysfunction. Only 2 boys had a full-scale IQ above 90. These uniquely vulnerable juveniles were unable to recognize the importance of psychiatric and neurologic symptoms to their defense. Their status was not fully appreciated at the time they were tried and sentenced.

▶ *These data are frightening. Not merely because of the horrible lives adolescents on "death row" have, but also because of our obvious inability as a society to effectively identify, treat, or prevent such victimization and its inevitable consequences. This is all the more reason to be as sensitive as possible to potential clues or hints of abuse in children seen for treatment of any kind.*

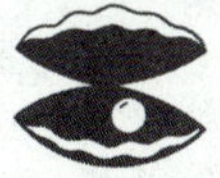

Pyromania is more commonly diagnosed in males; agoraphobia is more commonly diagnosed in females.

Addictive Disorders

Prevalence, Detection, and Treatment of Alcoholism in Hospitalized Patients

Moore RD, Bone LR, Geller G, et al
JAMA 261:403–407, Jan 20, 1989 **4–22**

How many alcholics would you expect to find when screening all new admissions to adult inpatient services? At Johns Hopkins Hospital fully 25% of medical and surgical patients and nearly 33% of psychiatric admissions were alcoholic. The lowest rate, for ob/gyn patients, was a not inconsiderable 12.5%. Except for psychiatric patients, fewer than half of the screen-positive individuals were detected by house staff and faculty physicians. The extent of intervention correlated with reported changes in alcohol use after discharge from the hospital. The most important message: Alcoholism must be sought far beyond the stereotypical "street alcoholic."

▶ *Physicians across all hospital services overlook alcohol abuse. They are especially blind when patients deny drinking, are women, or come from high educational or socioeconomic backgrounds. The most troublesome part is that if physicians don't intervene, patients don't change.*

Alcohol Consumption and Withdrawal in New-Onset Seizures

Ng SKC, Hauser WA, Brust JCM, et al
N Engl J Med 319:666–673, Sept 15, 1988 **4–23**

The precise role of alcohol excess per se and of alcohol withdrawal in inducing seizures is not clear. A case-control study included 300 subjects with seizures and an unmatched control group. Seizures not related to some event such as recent stroke increased with the alcohol intake, particularly at levels of 200 to 300 g daily. In provoked seizures, alcohol was a factor only when 200 g per day were taken. Close analysis of the timing of seizures showed that withdrawal from alcohol did not cause them. Most, if not all, alcohol-related seizures result from persistent excessive consumption.

▶ *When I was trained, the experts asserted that there was no such thing as "rum fits"; rather, seizures in alcoholics were believed to be the result of alcohol withdrawal. Well, here we come full circle: They are the result of alcohol, and they're dose related, and patients should be so informed.*

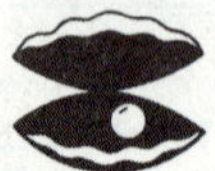

One third of Americans abstain from alcohol, but 10% of drinkers consume 50% of the alcohol.

Desipramine Facilitation of Initial Cocaine Abstinence

Gawin FH, Kleber HD, Byck R, et al
Arch Gen Psychiatry 46:117–121, February 1989 **4–24**

Both desipramine and lithium were compared with placebo in a double-blind 6-week trial in 70 cocaine abusers. Only desipramine substantially decreased the use of cocaine; lithium was not significantly better than placebo. Desipramine lowered the craving for cocaine and appears to be an effective first-line approach to those actively dependent on the drug. Desipramine may act by reversing cocaine-induced neuroadaptations and accelerating CNS normalization after a long period of abuse.

▶ *Cocaine represents a blight in America today, and any treatment that's effective is a blessing. Desipramine does not cure the addiction, but it does reduce craving and increases abstinence. As the authors are quick to point out, this is just the first step; it doesn't predict longer term abstinence, but it's a start.*

Cessation of Illicit Drug Use in Young Adulthood

Kandel DB, Raveis VH
Arch Gen Psychiatry 46:109–116, February 1989 **4–25**

The use of illicit drugs is strongly related to age. In 1,200 young adults surveyed, the factors predicting cessation of substance use in adulthood paralleled those that predicted freedom from abuse in adolescence: conventional social role performance, a social setting unfavorable to drug use, and good health. Past involvement with both legal and illicit drugs was a very important predictor, especially of marijuana use. With cocaine, use by friends was a prominent factor. Young adults who use illicit drugs chiefly for social reasons are more likely to stop than those who use them for personal enjoyment or for psychological reasons.

▶ *Adolescents stop taking drugs for the same reasons they never start, and assuming adult family responsibilities is an important force. The finding that those who take drugs because their peers do stop more often gives hope to methods of intervening; those taking them for psychological reasons are tougher to treat.*

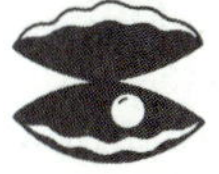

Marijuana is the most widely abused illegal drug in the United States.

Comparing Tobacco Cigarette Dependence With Other Drug Dependencies: Greater or Equal "Difficulty Quitting" and "Urges to Use," But Less "Pleasure" From Cigarettes

Kozlowski LT, Wilkinson A, Skinner W, et al
JAMA 261:898–901, Feb 10, 1989 **4–26**

What's hardest to quit: smoking, drinking, or using drugs? A majority of 1,000 alcohol and drug abusers thought that it would be harder to quit cigarettes than their problem substance. The urge to smoke was especially strong in those dependent on alcohol. Cigarettes generally were thought of as less pleasurable than alcohol or other drugs. Although smoking has declined in the general population, it remains prevalent in substance abusers. The other side of the coin is that heavy smokers are more likely than nonsmokers to have another substance problem.

▸ *Some people laughed when former Surgeon General Koop said that tobacco addiction was stronger than other kinds, but among substance abusers, it was judged tougher to kick. Ironically, as the rate of smoking decreases it appears that the hard-core residua will consist of persons addicted to multiple substances— e.g., alcohol, drugs, and tobacco.*

Long-Term Use of Nicotine Chewing Gum: Occurrence, Determinants, and Effect on Weight Gain

Hajek P, Jackson P, Belcher M
JAMA 260:1593–1596, Sept 16, 1988 **4–27**

Nicotine chewing gum can help smokers to stop, but what if they get hooked on the gum? Of about 500 clients of a smokers' clinic who received 2-mg nicotine gum, 34—a fourth of all abstainers—still used it a year later. Those who stopped smoking used the gum for 6 months on average, twice the recommended time. Long-term gum use did seem to minimize weight gain by abstainers. Nicotine gum does not create dependence on nicotine; it merely transfers it. It may well be that, without the gum, many persons would revert to smoking, and there is no question that chewing is a lesser evil.

▶ *A patient of mine asked for nicotine gum to help him stop smoking but immediately decided not to stop because of the increased boost the extra nicotine gave him. Granted, he may represent less than a quarter of the "successes," but it's still troubling. Nicotine gum is better than smoking, but we've got a way to go.*

Pathological Gambling: A Psychobiological Study

Roy A, Adinoff B, Roehrich L, et al
Arch Gen Psychiatry 45:369–373, April 1988 **4–28**

Noradrenergic function was assessed in pathologic gamblers as a special case of impulsiveness. In 24 patients, most with a lifetime diagnosis of affective disorder, plasma levels of the norepinephrine metabolite MHPG were increased, as was the centrally produced fraction of cerebrospinal fluid MHPG. The urinary output of norepinephrine also was higher in gamblers than in conrols. Gamblers who were depressed tended to have higher levels of diazepam-binding inhibitor in the cerebrospinal fluid. The findings suggest a disordered noradrenergic system in pathologic gamblers.

▶ *Gambling has represented one of the most neglected and least understood addictive behaviors. The finding that these patients' biologic abnormalities resemble those of sensation-seeking individuals, rather than those who are impulsive, may sound "academic," but it will lead to efforts to decrease such sensation seeking through psychological intervention and to further attempts to investigate the biologic mechanisms.*

Psychopharmacology

The Effect of Long-Term Treatment With Clozapine in Schizophrenia: A Retrospective Study in 96 Patients Treated With Clozapine for up to 13 Years

Lindström LH
Acta Psychiatr Scand 77:524–529, 1988 **4–29**

Treatment for a year or more with the dibenzodiazepine clozapine was tried in 76 schizophrenic and schizoaffective patients after neuroleptic therapy had proved ineffective or was unduly toxic. In more than a third of the patients clozapine was superior to past neuroleptic therapy. Even better, tolerance did not develop in responsive patients. Agranulocytosis developed in 1 patient and 4 had grand mal seizures, but there were no extrapyramidal side effects. The risk of side effects notwithstanding, alternatives to neuroleptic therapy must be tried in severely schizophrenic patients who are resistant to conventional treatment.

▶ *For more than 35 years we have had essentially the same medications available for the treatment of schizophrenia. For patients who did not respond, we could add lithium or carbamazapine, but there was no other fallback. Now clozapine has been shown to be effective and, despite its lethal side effects, will be used with treatment-resistant patients under a strict protocol. Good news indeed!*

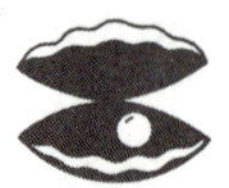

Van Gogh has been given several possible diagnoses, including schizophrenia, alcoholism, digitalis intoxication (the yellow vision affecting his painting), epilepsy, and bipolar disease.

Dose of Fluphenazine, Familial Expressed Emotion, and Outcome in Schizophrenia: Results of a Two-Year Controlled Study

Hogarty GE, McEvoy JP, Munetz M, et al
Arch Gen Psychiatry 45:797–805, September 1988 **4–30**

A 2-year controlled dose study of maintenance fluphenazine therapy was conducted in 70 recently discharged schizophrenic patients. Stabilized patients were assigned to receive either the same standard dose or 20% of the prescribed dose, which averaged 3.8 mg every 2 weeks. Relapse rates were unrelated to either dosage or level of expressed emotion. Side effects were less frequent in the low-dose group, and over time these patients had better interpersonal relationships than those given the standard dose. Patients with lower levels of expressed emotion were better adjusted. It would be interesting to learn whether psychosocial interventions are more effective in patients given low-dose maintenance medication.

▶ *This study has astounding implications—that low-dose regimens of maintenance fluphenazine result in better outcomes for patients with schizophrenia than standard doses do. We have to start lowering the doses of psychotropic medications, especially in patients who must take them for long periods of time.*

No Help From Lithium? About Patients Who Might Have Been But Were Not Helped by Prophylactic Lithium Treatment

Schou M
Comp Psychiatry 29:83–90, March–April 1988 **4–31**

Lithium sometimes is prescribed for those unlikely to benefit. More often, it is not given to those who probably would respond. Some patients for whom lithium is prescribed fail to comply with treatment or drop out for various reasons. The psychologist, nurse, social worker, and laboratory technician all can help to insure compliance with treatment. The best results can be expected if the dose is high enough to prevent relapse, but at the same time low enough to minimize adverse drug effects. The full prophylactic effect may require 6 to 12 months. If patients fail to respond in this time or do not tolerate lithium, other means of prophylaxis should be considered.

▶ *Mogens Schou, the Danish dean of lithium treatment, summarizes the largely nonpharmacologic reasons why lithium does not prevent recurrence of manic-depressive episodes. The lesson to be learned from this dissertation is that if lithium therapy is not even tried or isn't working, we'd better look into the reasons, because carefully titrated, long-term administration should do the trick.*

Treatment Guidelines for Psychotropic Drug Use in Pregnancy

Cohen LS, Heller VL, Rosenbaum JF
Psychosomatics 30:25–33, Winter 1989 **4–32**

It almost goes without saying that psychotropic drugs should be given to pregnant women only when the maternal and fetal risks of disease exceed those of treatment. Planned pregnancy obviously is important for patients already receiving these drugs. Sudden withdrawal of antipsychotic drugs can itself be hazardous. When psychosis develops during pregnancy, organic causes must be carefully excluded. Secondary amines such as nortriptyline and desipramine are the preferred antidepressants for use in pregnancy. The issue of breast-feeding must be addressed, because all psychotropic drugs are secreted in the milk.

▶ *Although we strive not to prescribe psychotropic medications in pregnant women, sometimes we have to. If we're forced to, however, we should rule out organicity, use small doses, use high-potency neuroleptics, and remember that all psychotropic drugs appear in the mother's milk. Lithium is the most teratogenic and the one we all usually stop.*

Other Psychiatric Treatment Issues

Mental Patients' Attitudes Toward Hospitalization: A Neglected Aspect of Hospital Tenure

Drake RE, Wallach MA
Am J Psychiatry 145:29–34, January 1988 **4–33**

Surely, it's appropriate to consider whether mental patients prefer continuing to live in the hospital over residing in the community. In a series of nearly 200 chronically ill patients in a state hospital aftercare program, patients' preferences strongly predicted both rehospitalization and total time in the hospital during 1 year of follow-up. Clinicians considered where the patient felt most comfortable and seemed to want to live. Not only can patient preferences help to explain certain conflicting results in studies of hospital tenure, but taking notice of the patient's perspective will make discharge planning more rational.

▶ *It sounds so obvious—if patients don't want to be in the hospital, their stays will be shorter and they'll avoid readmission. It's important to ask about their attitudes. Once again, we're reminded to go to the source when we want accurate information—to our patients and their families—rather than assume anything.*

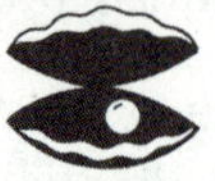

Nineteenth century medical textbooks claimed that masturbation lead to blindness and insanity.

A Randomized Clinical Trial of Inpatient Family Intervention: III. Effects at 6-Month and 18-Month Follow-Ups

Spencer JH Jr, Glick ID, Haas GL, et al
Am J Psychiatry 145:1115–1121, September 1988 **4–34**

Family intervention was integrated with medication and other measures for 169 psychiatric patients and the effects examined after 6 months and 18 months. Global functioning was better with family treatment at 6 months. At 18 months, females with schizophrenia or major affective disorder who received family treatment showed positive effects on all individual measures. In contrast, males with these diagnoses did not benefit from added family therapy. In some instances, family treatment appears to alter family attitudes, and this in turn can improve the patient's outcome.

▶ *For years we've assumed that a good inpatient program should include family therapy along with medication, psychotherapy, activities therapy, and so on. But we have had no data. Now we have, and we can justify family therapy for females with psychotic illnesses. But why males show no difference is puzzling.*

Empathy: Misconceptions and Misuses in Psychotherapy

Book HE
Am J Psychiatry 145:420–424, April 1988 **4–35**

Empathy, whereby a therapist comes to know and comprehend what the patient is experiencing consciously or unconsciously, is an essential therapeutic tool, but it often is misunderstood. The term refers to a way of gathering information about another person's internal experience, not to how it is used. Empathy is not sympathy, kindness, or approval. Although empathy is being able to finish a patient's sentence, doing so is often felt by the patient to be intrusive or infantilizing. The therapist must guard against using empathy defensively to gratify his own needs. Empathy is incorrectly used when the therapist disregards what's most important to the patient, wherein some things are much more important than others. It also is misused when a patient, though understood, feels damaged rather than comforted.

▶ *Truly understanding the patient is quite different from unquestioning acceptance, overidentification, "humoring the patient," or countertransferentially misusing empathy. The author employs the definition of empathy best when he states that it is being able to finish the patient's sentence but* not *doing it.*

Geropsychiatry

Bedside Differentiation of Depressive Pseudodementia From Dementia

Reynolds CF III, Hoch CC, Kupfer DJ, et al
Am J Psychiatry 145:1099–1103, September 1988 **4–36**

Older patients with features of both depression and dementia can be a difficult treatment problem. In comparing 28 patients with primary degenerative dementia and 14 with depressive pseudodementia, the latter had better Mini-Mental State scores and were less impaired on the Blessed dementia scale. Hamilton scores of depression were higher than in the demented group. Pseudodemented patients were more likely to be anxious and to have markedly impaired libido. Those who were demented tended to be disoriented in time and had trouble dressing themselves and finding their way about. It still is not certain whether coexisting cognitive impairment and major depression are preludes to progressive dementing illness.

▶ *To propertly treat the elderly who appear demented, one must differentiate dementia from depression masquerading as dementia. The bottom line here is that patients with depressive pseudodementia have more early morning awakening, psychological anxiety, and loss of libido, and patients with "true" dementia have more disorientation to time, difficulty in finding their way about inside or outside, and greater difficulty with dressing.*

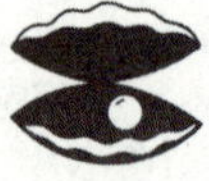

Any patient taking antipsychotics who becomes feverish should be assessed for malignant neuroleptic syndrome.

The Development and Initial Validation of a Sensitive Bedside Cognitive Screening Test

Faust D, Fogel BS
J Nerv Ment Dis 177:25–31, January 1989 **4–37**

The High Sensitivity Cognitive Screen (HSCS) is designed to detect more subtle cognitive deficits than the Mini-Mental State Examination and is just as sensitive and efficient. It is a 20-minute interview-based test. Most items are adapted for bedside use from standard neuropsychological tests. Test-retest and interrater reliability was adequate. In a series of 60 psychiatric and neurologic patients, using formal neuropsychological testing as the standard, the HSCS correctly classified 93% of subjects as normal or abnormal.

▶ *Another problem with the elderly is detecting early or subtle organicity. The authors' new assessment sounds much more sensitive than the Mini-Mental State Exam, the usual standard. The problem is that, although they describe it, they don't publish it or tell you how to purchase it.*

Prevalence, Frequency, and Duration of Hypnotic Drug Use Among the Elderly Living at Home

Morgan K, Dallosso H, Ebrahim S, et al
Br Med J 296:601–602, Feb 27, 1988 **4–38**

Long-term hypnotic drug use by elderly persons can lead to confusion, psychomotor impairment, increased anxiety, and even rebound insomnia. Of 1,000 randomly selected persons aged 65 or more, 16% reported using hypnotics, chiefly benzodiazepines. Also, about 75% of users had taken the drugs for longer than a year and 25% for more than 10 years. The most frequently prescribed drug was nitrazepam. Many elderly users of hypnotic drugs are unnecessarily exposed to the effects of drug accumulation, daytime withdrawal reactions, or benzodiazepine dependence.

▶ *A recent report, featured prominently on front pages of most newspapers, focused on the widespread mega- and poly-pharmacy practiced in many nursing homes. This report concentrates on prescribed drugs taken at home. We all must be careful not to encourage the long-*

term use of benzodiazepines, especially the long-acting ones, because of their severe cumulative effects.

Clinical Issues

Why Patients Multilate Themselves

Favazza AR
Hosp Community Psychiatry 40:137–145, February 1989 **4–39**

Patients with a wide range of psychiatric disorders attempt to destroy or alter their body tissues without consciously attempting suicide. The spectrum of this behavior ranges from self-cutting and hitting to enucleation or the amputation of limbs or genitals. Excepting several retarded patients and some of those with "organic" disorders, self-mutilation is best viewed as a purposeful, if morbid, attempt at self-help. The physician must try to deal as equably with self-mutilators as with those who are suicidal.

▶ *For most medical students, the most disturbing and unbelievable symptoms exhibited by psychiatric patients involve self-mutilation. Trying to find a common theme, given the varieties of symptoms, diagnoses, and patient explanations, is nearly impossible. The teaching point of this paper, unfortunately, has to be that each individual's symptom must be explored and even then the explanation may be conjectural.*

Splitting Schizophrenia

Lander ES
Nature 336:105–106, Nov 10, 1988 **4–40**

After 80 years, no accepted cause of schizophrenia and indeed no unifying concept exist. The field remains open to all, most prominently the geneticists. Sherrington et al. (*Nature* 336:164–167, 1988) have reported that in 5 Icelandic and 2 English families comprising 39 cases (all of the major subtypes included), schizophrenia was coinherited with a region on the long arm of chromosome 5. At the same time, Kennedy et al. (*Nature* 336:167–170, 1988), studying a large Swedish family, refuted this finding. What steered researchers in this direction was the report of a schizophrenic uncle and nephew who each had an extra copy of 5q11-13 translocated onto chromosome 1. Even if this locus proves not to be important, it is the first step in categorizing patients genetically and as such may help in assessing potential treatments. The best approach might be to map the genetic basis for the atypical physiologic or biochemical responses found in some schizophrenics rather than attempting to map the disease itself.

▶ *When word of a genetic marker on chromosome 5 in schizophrenia hit the newspapers, it was greeted with great anticipatory excitement. Although previous links had been established in families with affective disorders, no such thing had been done in schizophrenia. The fact that not all families have this same finding is further evidence that schizophrenia is a multi-etiologic disease or diseases.*

Schizophrenic Thought Disorder: A Psychological and Organic Interpretation

Cutting J, Murphy D
Br J Psychiatry 152:310–319, March 1988 **4–41**

In addition to dyslogia, delusional content, and disordered expression of thought, many schizophrenics are deficient in the way they think about or judge events in the real world: They display a true lack of common sense. When 20 subacute and chronic schizophrenic patients had their practical and social knowledge assessed, the lack of such knowledge proved to be the most prevalent form of thought disorder. What's more, it is independent of the other manifestations.

▶ *When we in the United States speak of thought disorders in schizophrenia, we are usually referring to looseness of associations. This report from England, however, hones in on the lack of "common sense." This deficit is not found exclusively in schizophrenia, but it is a good way of assessing whether someone may have it.*

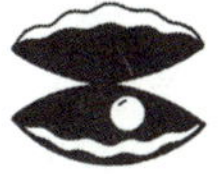

The more atypical the symptom course, the more the physician should entertain the diagnosis of organic motor disorder and factitious disorder.

A Neuroanatomical Hypothesis for Panic Disorder

Gorman JM, Liebowitz MR, Fyer AJ, et al
Am J Psychiatry 146:148–161, February 1989 **4–42**

A neuroanatomical model could reconcile prevailing views of panic disorder as a biologic or a psychological disease. Acute panic attacks are related to excitation in the brain stem, anticipatory anxiety to the limbic system, and phobic avoidance behavior to the prefrontal cortex. Antipanic drugs such as imipramine and phenelzine block brain-stem-provoked panic attacks. Relaxation techniques and benzodiazepines lower anticipatory anxiety, and densensitization and cognitive approaches relieve phobic avoidance. This model neither contradicts nor validates psychodynamic formulations of panic disorder.

▶ *Although clearly labeled a hypothesis, the authors' view of anatomical loci for specific aspects of panic disorders is worthy of consideration and investigation. This will constitute an enormous step forward if it can be confirmed.*

The Northwick Park "Functional" Psychosis Study: Diagnosis and Treatment Response

Johnstone EC, Crow TJ, Frith CD, et al
Lancet 2:119–125, July 16, 1988 **4–43**

Treatment response is taken as a criterion validating the diagnosis of schizophrenia or manic-depressive psychosis. Nevertheless, in a trial of more than 120 functionally psychotic patients, the dopamine antagonist neuroleptic drug pimozide relieved hallucinations, delusions, and incongruity of affect, regardless of mood elevation or depression. The only real effect of lithium was to lower elevated mood. These findings suggest that it may make more sense to view functional psychosis as a continuum rather than categorizing it into distinct schizophrenic and manic-depressive illnesses.

▶ *The argument about whether we have one (psychotic) mental illness or several has raged for years. The authors, yet mindful that recent findings of genetic loci for specific diseases (above 40) would destroy the one-disease theory, believe that their study supports it. Who knows?*

5

Surgery

Pharmacodynamics of Antibiotic Penetration of Tissue and Surgical Prophylaxis

Bergamini TM, Polk HC Jr
Surg Gynecol Obstet 168:283–289, March 1989 **5–1**

The key to preventing surgical infection is to make sure that an adequate level of antibiotic is present in the tissues throughout the procedure. All of the factors that make up the pharmacokinetics of antibiotic distribution and excretion come into play. A drug with a longer serum half-life is more active for a longer time than others, but limiting the duration of postoperative prophylaxis to 24 hours or less will reduce the number of drug-associated complications. Theory aside, clinical trials are required to learn how long a given antibiotic prevents postoperative infection.

▸ *One of the problems confronting physicians is making an antibiotic selection based on a rational appreciation of the properties of the given drug rather than on the polemics of a drug retail salesman. So many antibiotics are currently available that it is difficult to remember not only their names but also their targets. The best advice is to limit the number of drugs you use so that you'll have a complete appreciation of each medication's effects.*

Metabolic Response to Sepsis and Trauma

Douglas RG, Shaw JHF
Br J Surg 76:115–122, February 1989 **5–2**

Neuroendocrine responses and inflammatory mediators released from the local wound or septic focus both contribute to the metabolic response to trauma and sepsis. The most prominent hormones released are epinephrine, glucagon, and cortisol; interleukin 1 released by damaged tissue may accelerate proteolysis in surgical patients. The turnover of glucose is more rapid, but glucose also is oxidized less efficiently. Fat is apparently the preferred energy substrate, at least in septic patients. Adequate substrate and nitrogen may not reduce the catabolic response itself, but they do promote protein synthesis, thereby lowering net catabolism. A current question: Will growth hormone prove therapeutically useful?

▶ *Current work on septic shock focuses on the mediators that produce injury and tissue damage as well as the symptoms. Specific antibodies to recombinant human mediators can be produced. Cachectin has been identified as a proximate mediator of the shock and tissue injury induced by lipopolysaccharide. Monoclonal antibody blockage of cachectin can prevent all the effects of the injection of endotoxin or live* Escherichia coli *organisms. Maintenance of nitrogen balance with intravenous fluids alone cannot reverse cellular injury from starvation. The closing statement, "To date, the clinical efficacy of none [no substrate, or hormonal or pharmacologic manipulation] has been conclusively proved," is extremely revealing.*

The Gut: A Central Organ After Surgical Stress

Wilmore DW, Smith RJ, O'Dwyer ST, et al
Surgery 104:917–923, November 1988 **5–3**

The gut traditionally is viewed as being inactive, or quiescent, in injured or infected patients. But recent studies of intestinal exchange based on portal venous sampling suggest that the gut has a significant metabolic role under conditions of fasting and stress. By using glutamine the gut mucosa spares glucose, but glutamine deficiency can lead to mucosal atrophy. Early and adequate provision of glutamine in the diet promotes intestinal cellularity and helps maintain the barrier function of the gut. An alternative: parenteral feedings containing glutamine.

▶ *In the past the intestine was regarded as a passive element in surgical stress, but it now is believed to play a critical role. The implications of early enteral feeding to obviate some of the adverse effects of stress and the role of glutamine undoubtedly has significant clinical implications. Although we had passed through a phase in which parenteral feeding was used much too liberally and the pendulum has swung away from it, this change in attitude should not pertain to truly stressed patients.*

Thin Stage I Primary Cutaneous Malignant Melanoma: Comparison of Excision With Margins of 1 or 3 cm

Veronesi U, Cascinelli N, Adamus J, et al
N Engl J Med 318:1159–1162, May 5, 1988 **5–4**

How much normal skin should be taken when a primary melanoma is removed? Groups of 300 patients with melanomas no thicker than 2 mm had either narrow excision with 1-cm margins or wide excision with margins of 3 cm or more. All 3 patients whose initial relapse took the form of local recurrence had undergone narrow excision. Nevertheless, no significant differences in regional node metastases, distant metastases, or survival were noted. Skin-sparing narrow excision is as effective as conventional wide excision in patients with cutaneous melanoma no thicker than 2 mm.

▶ *This definitive article demonstrates that early thin melanoma is curable. A narrow excision is a safe procedure. The authors emphasize the importance of distinguishing melanoma by thickness and fashioning the therapeutic regimen accordingly. The policy of selecting the excision for cutaneous malignant melanoma is actually a recent chapter in surgery.*

The Tension-Free Hernioplasty

Lichtenstein IL, Shulman AG, Amid PK, et al
Am J Surg 157:188–193, February 1989 **5–5**

Half a million groin hernia repairs are done each year in the United States, as many as one fifth because of recurrent inguinal hernia. Marlex, a polypropylene, is an ideal material for permanently reinforcing hernial defects. A sheet of polypropylene mesh is secured medially to the lacunar ligament, laterally along Poupart's ligament, and superiorly to the rectus sheath and conjoined muscle and tendon. None of the most recent 1,000 consecutive patients treated had recurrence. Infection is not a problem when antimicrobial powder is sprinkled into the surgical wound. Often, patients can do manual labor within 2 or 3 days of surgery.

▶ *The concept presented in this paper is a complete switch from the classic approach to inguinal hernia. The distinction between congenital hernias and acquired hernias is significant, and we currently believe that sewing together the edges of acquired hernias leads to a high recurrence rate. Application of the patch and avoidance of tension are reasonable considerations, and the reported negligible recurrence rate has not been achieved by any other technique. Among those surgeons who dedicate their practices to the management of hernia, this approach has been widely accepted.*

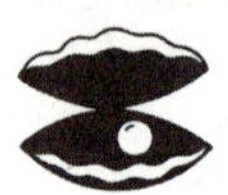

More than a half million deaths from coronary heart disease occur each year. The state with the highest attack rate is New York with 303 deaths per 100,000 population; the lowest is Hawaii with 166 per 100,000. We'll let you draw your own conclusions.

Surgical Treatment of Graves' Disease

Ozoux JP, de Calan L, Portier G, et al
Am J Surg 156:177–181, September 1988 **5–6**

In Graves' disease the thyroid is victim of an immunologic conflict, the origin of which is poorly understood. In a surgical series of 88 patients, the most common indications were recurrence after medical therapy and a large or hypervascular goiter. There were no postoperative deaths, and no patient experienced permanent hypoparathyroidism. Two patients had temporary dysphonia caused by the surgery. Hyperthyroidism recurred in 15 patients, whereas 12 had hypothyroidism. It would be nice to have both few recurrences and infrequent hypothyroidism, but this is a pipe dream! It is better to treat postoperative hypothyroidism than to have to deal with recurrent Graves' disease.

▶ *The treatment of Graves' disease by thyroidectomy remains controversial. It generally is agreed that operation is indicated when the gland is large and causes tracheal compression, when medical therapy fails, in some pregnant women, or because of patient choice. It is difficult to decide what the remnant size should be. The important point made in this article is that effective thyroidectomy cannot be defined at the time of hospital discharge. This relates to both thyroid and parathyroid function.*

Ductal Carcinoma In Situ (Intraductal Carcinoma) of the Breast

Schnitt SJ, Silen W, Sadowsky NL, et al
N Engl J Med 318:898–902, Apr 7, 1988 **5–7**

Intraductal carcinoma now accounts for as many as one fifth of breast cancers in mammographic screening series. Apart from a small mammographic focus, intraductal carcinoma can be detected as an incidental lesion, with nipple discharge, or as a palpable mass of any size. In some patients having biopsy alone, invasive cancer will develop. Mastectomy is standard treatment for in situ ductal carcinoma. The risk of local recurrence probably is greater with breast-conserving surgery no matter how carefully patients are selected, and half of those with local recurrence will have invasive disease. Preliminary data suggest that radiotherapy can reduce, or at least delay, local recurrence.

▸ *Because of the widespread use of mammography this diagnosis is being made with increasing frequency. The authors provide a complete assessment of the situation and present the results of various forms of treatment in appropriate fashion. It needs to be stressed, however, that the median follow-up period for the excision and radiotherapy and for the excision alone series is about 4 years.*

Breast Cancer in Women After Augmentation Mammoplasty

Silverstein MJ, Handel N, Gamagami P, et al
Arch Surg 123:681–685, June 1988 **5–8**

A million American women have had augmentation mammoplasty; breast cancer has developed, or will do so, in 1 of every 10. In a 5-year period 20 such patients had infiltrating cancer that was first detected as a palpable mass. Two thirds of these patients had node disease and, more to the point, none of the cancers was occult. In contrast, 1 in 5 cancers in patients without augmentation mammoplasty were occult. A silicone gel implant makes film-screen mammography less sensitive. Consequently, patients who have had augmentation mammoplasty and are older than age 35 years should have mammography annually, and all palpable lesions and mammographic abnormalities should be biopsied.

▶ *A series of articles have reported that breast reconstruction after mastectomy does not interfere with early detection of local recurrence in the operative site. However, few articles deal with breast cancer in patients after augmentation mammoplasty. Because of the difficulty in detecting breast cancer in a breast augmented with an implant, implantation should not be performed in high-risk patients with a strong family history of breast carcinoma.*

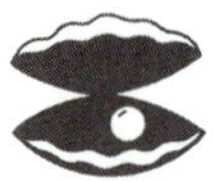

Remember this with regard to peripheral vascular surgery: One operation per patient per day.—John Bergan, M.D., Northwestern University, Chicago

A Randomized Clinical Trial Evaluating Tamoxifen in the Treatment of Patients With Node-Negative Breast Cancer Who Have Estrogen-Receptor-Positive Tumors

Fisher B, Costantino J, Redmond C, et al
N Engl J Med 320:479–484, Feb 23, 1989 **5–9**

Tamoxifen in a dosage of 10 mg twice daily was tested in more than 2,500 women with estrogen-receptor-positive breast cancers and negative axillary nodes. After 4 years no overall survival advantage was indicated, but disease-free survival was prolonged in tamoxifen-treated patients, especially those younger than 50 years of age. Treatment failure, recurrence, and tumor in the other breast all occurred less often with tamoxifen therapy, and toxicity was minimal. This is clearly a situation in which moderate benefit in clinical trials could translate into a substantial public health boon.

▶ *A series of randomized clinical trials shepherded by Dr. Fisher and his associates has finally provided us with meaningful data that allow surgeons to act intelligently. The low incidence of side effects associated with tamoxifen would suggest that there is no reason not to use it in this category of patients. A 4-year survival rate of more than 90% in all patients is what we would anticipate with a histologically negative axillary node. The significant difference in the disease-free interval is encouraging. It would be interesting to follow these patients as far as*

10 years postoperatively to see if any survival advantage has been realized with the use of tamoxifen.

Effects of Adjuvant Tamoxifen and of Cytotoxic Therapy on Mortality in Early Breast Cancer: An Overview of 61 Randomized Trials Among 28,896 Women

Early Breast Cancer Trialists' Collaborative Group
N Engl J Med 319:1681–1692, Dec 29, 1988 **5–10**

Worldwide mortality data for early breast cancer with or without regional node involvement covered 16,500 women in 28 trials of tamoxifen and nearly 13,500 others in 40 chemotherapy trials; approximately 4,000 deaths occurred in each group. Tamoxifen clearly lowered 5-year mortality in women aged 50 years and older. Chemotherapy reduced mortality only in women younger than 50 years of age. Combination chemotherapy was better than single-drug treatment. It may not be necessary to continue chemotherapy for longer than 4–6 months. The question remains: How relevant are these observations to the long-term survival of women treated for early breast cancer?

▶ *This extraordinary study provides meaningful data demonstrating the efficacy of tamoxifen and cytotoxic therapy in reducing mortality. It is only through studies such as this that involve randomized trials and incorporate the collaborative efforts of many groups that true answers can be achieved. Such an approach is one of the major contributions of modern scientific medicine.*

Early Experience With the Total Artificial Heart as a Bridge to Cardiac Transplantation

Copeland JG, Smith RG, Icenogle TB, et al
Surg Clin North Am 68:621–634, June 1988 **5–11**

In the past 2 decades 80 artificial hearts (orthotopic biventricular pneumatic pulsatile artificial devices) were implanted, usually with the goal of maintaining a critically ill patient until transplantation was feasible. However, 5 implants were "permanent." Of 49 patients who received cardiac transplants, 33 are alive. Concern over excessive bleeding, embolism, and infection has been allayed to a substantial degree. The device does provide excellent and immediate circulatory control. After 3 weeks, however, the risks of infection and marked scar tissue reaction become considerable, and this currently is the outer time limit of support.

▶ *This article provides the synopsis of the total world experience with the artificial heart. There is little question that the role of the artificial heart is that of a temporizing device for a patient awaiting transplantation. It is appropriate to continue efforts to improve technology in light of the problems associated with the availability of donor hearts.*

Selective Use of Extracorporeal Membrane Oxygenation in the Management of Congenital Diaphragmatic Hernia

Stolar C, Dillon P, Reyes C
J Pediatr Surg 23:207–211, March 1988 **5–12**

When infants with congenital diaphragmatic hernia deteriorate, extracorporeal membrane oxygenation (ECMO) provides rest for the lungs. Fourteen such infants who appeared at first to have adequate lung parenchyma were placed on ECMO for 2–9 days; 12 survived. Right-to-left shunting decreased during treatment in these infants. Whereas infants with overwhelming pulmonary hypoplasia do not respond to ECMO, those who otherwise would die primarily of pulmonary hypertension can be saved. Which infants are these? Those whose best predicted partial pressure of oxygen exceeds 100 torr and whose partial pressure of carbon dioxide is less than 50 torr with maximal treatment.

▶ *Although many indications for the use of ECMO have evolved, the most dramatic results have occurred in patients with congenital diaphragmatic hernia. When distinction is made between pulmonary hypoplasia and pulmonary hypertension in these newborns, that information provides meaningful criteria for selection. The use of ECMO is extremely labor intensive, and more accurate information about which patients would benefit from its use is welcome.*

Extracorporeal Membrane Oxygenation in Children: New Trends

Trento A, Thompson A, Siewers RD, et al
J Thorac Cardiovasc Surg 96:542–547, October 1988 **5–13**

Four fifths of 39 neonates recently treated by extracorporeal membrane oxygenation (ECMO) survived, compared with about half of 33 infants treated earlier. Total apneic lung rest now is used when pulmonary interstitial emphysema persists; 5 of 6 such neonates survived. Four of 7 patients treated for left ventricular or biventricular failure after cardiopulmonary bypass were long-term survivors. The benefits of ECMO far outweigh the risks in high-risk infants. Membrane oxygenation is the best approach to severe post-bypass left ventricular failure when the infant's lungs can be ventilated to obtain a carbon dioxide tension of 30 mm Hg and when use of other ventricular assist devices is not feasible.

▶ *Extracorporeal membrane oxygenation has been used with increasing frequency in newborns with severe respiratory failure. Recently, Zwischenberger et al. (J Pediatr Surg 23:599, 1988) reported that 9% of their patients had life-threatening intrathoracic complications requiring emergency intervention while on ECMO. They managed 3 patients with tension hemothorax, 2 with tension pneumothorax, and 2 with pericardial tamponade. Four patients required emergency thoracotomy for definitive treatment. All 7 patients were weaned from ECMO and are short-term survivors.*

"Maximal" Thymectomy for Myasthenia Gravis: Results

Jaretzki A III, Penn AS, Younger DS, et al
J Thorac Cardiovasc Surg 95:747–757, May 1988 **5–14**

Because thymic tissue is widely distributed in the neck and mediastinum, reliable removal requires an en bloc transcervical-transsternal thymectomy. Ninety-five patients with generalized myasthenia had a "maximal" operation. Of 72 patients without thymoma, 69 benefited. The remission rate at 7 years was 81%. Three of 8 other patients who were reexplored because of incapacitating weakness improved, as did 9 of 15 patients with thymoma. Two thymoma patients died in crisis. Thorough removal of thymus is called for in patients with generalized myasthenia and in those with thymoma, whether or not myasthenia gravis is present.

▶ *The authors emphasize that thymectomy remains an effective treatment for selected patients with myasthenia gravis. The preparation of patients with preoperative plasmapheresis has reduced significantly the complications associated with an operation. The need for the extensive operation championed in the present article is a subject of debate. Equally good results have been achieved with standard transsternal thymectomy. A small group of surgeons still indicate that they achieve equivalent results with transcervical thymectomy.*

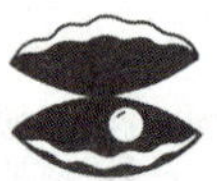

Toe swelling in association with a swollen leg usually means lymphedema.—John Bergan, M.D., Northwestern University, Chicago

Thrombolytic Therapy: Current Status

Marder VJ, Sherry S
N Engl J Med 318:1585–1595, June 16, 1988 **5–15**

The latest word in thrombolysis is regionalization, either by using agents that bind selectively to a thrombus or by infusing drugs into the occluded vessel. Fibrinolytic drugs undoubtedly accelerate vascular reperfusion, whether in an embolized pulmonary artery, a deep leg vein, or a stenotic, thrombosed peripheral vessel or coronary artery. Complexes of a thrombolytic drug, especially tissue plasminogen activator, and a monoclonal antibody hold promise. Chemical methods of extending the half-life of thrombolytic agents and of lessening their antigenicity are being examined. Thrombolytic treatment also may be combined with beta-blockers or antiplatelet drugs.

▶ *This is the second part of an article related to thrombolytic therapy. The possibility of providing regional therapy and the efficacy of thrombolytic therapy for the management of pulmonary embolism, deep venous thrombosis, peripheral arterial occlusion, and myocardial infarction have broad implications. The technique may reduce markedly the indication for angioplasty. It may also have an impact on the indications for surgical intervention. We don't yet know whether there is a preferred thrombolytic agent.*

Carotid Endarterectomy—A Crisis in Confidence

Hertzer NR

J Vasc Surg 7:611–619, May 1988 **5–16**

Many surgeons today are wary about carotid endarterectomy. Too little is known about the risk of this operation at community hospitals, where most of these operations actually are done. Most surgeons are aware that stroke is not inevitable in a patient with disease at the carotid bifurcation, even if endarterectomy is never done. Carotid endarterectomy may be a simple operation conceptually, but it is technically unforgiving, and most surgeons are themselves not certain about their own results. The answer lies in establishing the safety of endarterectomy in each hospital and applying the same standards across the community.

▶ *In most centers with a long-term interest and a significant caseload of carotid endarterectomies, the operative mortality and morbidity rates have been extremely low (range, 1% to 2%). In those centers a case can be made for the appropriateness of carotid endarterectomy in symptomatic patients. Those who are opposed to carotid endarterectomy and in favor of the use of antiplatelet aggregating agents defend their thesis with a referral to those series with higher mortality and morbidity rates. In those centers in which the mortality and morbidity rates are disproportionately high, carotid endarterectomy should not be as widely applicable.*

Intracranial Hemorrhage After Carotid Endarterectomy

Pomposelli FB, Lamparello PJ, Riles TS, et al

J Vasc Surg 7:248–255, February 1988 **5–17**

After 11 of 1,500 carotid endarterectomies, intracranial bleeding on the same side was noted within 10 days of surgery, and about one third of these patients died. Hemiparesis was the most frequent symptom, but 3 patients had seizures. Half of the patients had a systolic pressure of more than 200 mm Hg postoperatively. The only evident disposing factor was relief of carotid stenosis greater than 90%. None of the affected patients required a shunt, and all had normal coagulation studies. Close monitoring of blood pressure can prevent uncontrolled hypertension in this setting.

▶ *This is an important review focusing on a rare complication of carotid endarterectomy performed for the relief of high-grade stenosis or transient ischemic attacks. Monitoring for postoperative hypertension is important, and the hypertension should be controllable. I agree with the author that the routine use of shunts would in no way prevent this complication. Careful monitoring of the blood pressure and prevention of significant hypertension seem reasonable.*

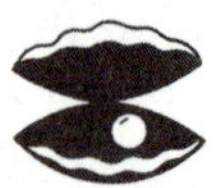

Patients with thalassemia major have shortened life spans. Surprisingly, the most common cause of death is heart disease, followed by infection, liver disease, and malignancy.

Percutaneous Transluminal Angioplasty Versus Operation for Peripheral Arteriosclerosis: Report of a Prospective Randomized Trial in a Selected Group of Patients

Wilson SE, Wolf GL, Cross AP
J Vasc Surg 9:1–9, January 1989 **5–18**

Clinically comparable groups of about 125 patients with occlusive disease in the iliac, superficial femoral, or popliteal arteries underwent surgical reconstruction or angioplasty. The immediate failure rate after angioplasty was 15%. During operation 1 death occurred, and 2 late deaths were ascribed to complications of surgery. After 5 years the numbers of major amputations and the level of clinical improvement were similar in the 2 groups. Angioplasty, when successful, seems as durable as surgery, and if it fails reconstruction still can be effective.

▶ *As is generally the case, the use of a prospective, randomized trial to assess the comparative value of 2 therapeutic approaches is indicated. Comparison of the 2 modalities of therapy certainly is appropriate for claudication-related iliac occlusion. A question can be raised about the assessment of patients who have claudication and femoral popliteal occlusion because, in general, surgery is not carried out for claudication alone unless it is severe. This study suggests that if percutaneous transluminal angioplasty (PCTA) and surgery yield comparable results, PCTA is preferred because of decreased cost and morbidity.*

Initial Results of Laser Recanalization in Lower Extremity Arterial Reconstruction

Seeger JM, Abela GS, Silverman JH, et al
J Vasc Surg 9:10–17, January 1989 **5–19**

Another in the lengthening list of laser applications: relief of total occlusions in the superficial femoral, popliteal, and common iliac arteries. Half of 46 patients treated with an argon laser had symptomatic relief and improved ankle-brachial indices. Only 1 patient required emergency surgical reconstruction after laser therapy failed, and none required treatment for perforation or bleeding. Half of the patients who had a good outcome would have been candidates for standard surgical treatment. Several others would not because of unacceptable medical or surgical risks.

▸ *This article was included because of the enthusiasm of those interested in surgical technology. The general sense is that, although it has been hoped that laser recanalization in lower extremity arterial reconstruction would obviate the need for bypass surgery and would reduce the hospital stay and morbidity, these improvements actually have occurred in only a relatively small percentage of patients. Laser energy is used, but what is actually effective is heat-probe coring of the thrombosis. Refinements of technique in the laser field are needed to achieve better results.*

Prevention of Venous Thromboembolism in General Surgical Patients: Results of Meta-Analysis

Clagett GP, Reisch JS
Ann Surg 208:227–240, August 1988 **5–20**

Active measures certainly are needed to prevent venous thromboembolism in patients having general surgery, but which are most effective? A survey of randomized clinical trials revealed that most prophylactic methods other than aspirin lower the rate of deep venous thrombosis, but only low-dose heparin and dextran clearly prevent pulmonary embolism. Heparin was better than dextran in preventing deep venous thrombosis, especially when administered every 8 hours. A risk of wound hematoma was noted, but major bleeding is not a problem.

▶ *This type of analysis is particularly important because each of the modalities considered has a series of articles extolling its virtues and another series of articles indicating its ineffectiveness. The 19% confirmed deep venous thrombosis rate reported for general surgical patients is extremely impressive. Our own experience suggests that clinically apparent deep venous thrombosis occurs less commonly.*

Resurrection of the *In Situ* Saphenous Vein Bypass: 1000 Cases Later

Leather RP, Shah DJ, Chang BB, et al
Ann Surg 208:435–442, October 1988 **5–21**

When limb-threatening ischemia is present the length and low flow rate of a distal bypass, whether a synthetic or a long free vein graft, often exceed functional limits. Use of the saphenous vein in place can provide a viable antithrombogenic endothelial flow surface. An in situ bypass was completed in 94% of 1,000 attempts using the valve incision technique. Two thirds of the bypasses extended below the infrapopliteal level. In more than half of the extremities the distal vein diameter was less than 3.5 mm. Nevertheless, 90% of the bypasses were patent after 1 year, and 76% were open at 5 years.

▶ *These authors were responsible for maintaining and rekindling interest in the use of the in situ saphenous vein bypass. There is little question that the use of a vein graft is clearly superior to the use of a prosthetic graft. Applying new methods to disrupt the valves has improved the procedure. A patency rate that includes 661 infrapopliteal bypasses is truly outstanding.*

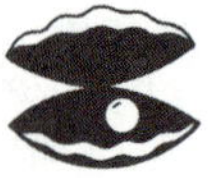

Each month, more than 25% of American children take prescription medication, and almost half of them take it incorrectly—either too much, too little, or for too short a time.

Valve Reconstruction Procedures for Nonobstructive Venous Insufficiency: Rationale, Techniques, and Results in 107 Procedures With Two- to Eight-Year Follow-up

Raju S, Fredericks R
J Vasc Surg 7:301–310, February 1988 **5–22**

In 200 extremities with nonobstructive chronic venous insufficiency, reflux in the deep venous system was the predominant condition. Superficial venous and perforator incompetence always was accompanied by deep reflux. Operations in 100 patients included valvuloplasty, axillary vein transfer, and wrapping of the valve with a Dacron sleeve. Most often, a redundant valve was coapted improperly. The need for stockings was less after surgery, and venous pressure measurements generally demonstrated improvement. Even modest improvement in postexercise pressure may be enough for stasis ulcers to heal.

▶ *This is a large series describing a procedure uncommonly performed by most vascular surgeons. Ferris and Kistner (*Arch Surg *117:1571, 1982) reviewed a 15-year experience with 53 femoral-venous reconstructions. Good to excellent results were obtained in about 80% of their patients. Johnson et al. (*Arch Surg *116:1461, 1981) reported that their experience with venous valve surgery provided less than favorable results. The discussion of this paper points out a series of patients in whom the perforating veins were not treated. The other expressed criticism has been that the test used to evaluate valvular incompetence, the Valsalva-induced foot pressure, correlated most closely with the operative results. It is believed that because this test was performed in the supine position, it bore little relationship to the severity of the physiologic aberration responsible for severe stasis changes.*

Twelve-Year Experience With the Greenfield Vena Caval Filter

Greenfield LJ, Michna BA
Surgery 104:706–712, October 1988 **5–23**

In 469 vena caval filter placements, the usual reasons for placement were contraindications to or failure of anticoagulation. Jugular placement was most common. Seven patients died of pulmonary thromboembolism within 48 hours of surgery, and 9 later deaths were ascribed to the same cause. Including 9 episodes of nonfatal embolism, the overall rate of recurrence was 4% in 12 years. All but 2% of the filters remained patent for the long term. More than 40% of patients had sequelae of venous stasis, but only 3% had ulceration. The suprarenal filter is an appropriate choice for young women planning a pregnancy.

▶ *Use of the Greenfield filter has become the standard technique for mechanical control of the cava to prevent pulmonary embolism. Certainly, heparin remains the keystone of therapeutic management of venous thrombosis in the prevention of pulmonary embolization. Failure of anticoagulation to prevent pulmonary emboli actually is an uncommon event. The use of a mechanical device such as the Greenfield filter is most commonly indicated when anticoagulation treatment is contraindicated.*

Pulmonary Embolectomy for Acute Massive Pulmonary Embolism: An Analysis of 71 Cases

Gray HH, Morgan JM, Paneth M, et al
Br Heart J 60:196–200, September 1988 **5–24**

A group of 71 patients underwent the removal of massive pulmonary emboli, experiencing marked hemodynamic compromise as a result. Of these 71, 25 sustained a significant period of cardiac arrest preoperatively. Two thirds of these patients but only 5 (11%) of the others died. Most patients who did survive had little morbidity. Only 1 patient required long-term anticoagulation, and only 2 had another embolism. Embolectomy certainly remains a viable option when thrombolysis is contraindicated or the patient is too ill.

▶ *Pulmonary embolism rarely leads to chronic pulmonary hypertension. Daily et al.* (J Thorac Cardiovasc Surg *93:221–233, 1987) describe bilateral pulmonary thromboendarterectomy with mediastinotomy, cardiopulmonary bypass, deep hypothermia, and circulatory arrest for relief of pulmonary hypertension caused by chronic pulmonary embolism; they report their experience with this technique in 41 patients. Myocardial preservation with cooling of the right and left ventricles and avoidance of entrance into the pleural space during dissection of the pulmonary arteries achieved the best hospital mortality rate.*

Major Blunt Abdominal Trauma Due to Child Abuse

Cooper A, Floyd T, Barlow B, et al
J Trauma 28:1483–1487, October 1988 **5–25**

Approximately half of abused children with blunt abdominal injuries die. The 22 patients treated at 2 centers in a 15-year period make up less than 0.5% of all abused children treated at those centers. Only 2 families were intact, and here the child was abused by a sitter. Overall, mortality was 45%. Of 6 children in profound shock from massive bleeding, 5 died; 4 others were dead on arrival. More of these children survive only if prompt care is possible. Immediate aggressive surgery is called for if hypovolemic shock or peritonitis is present.

▶ *This situation demands an appreciation of the widespread nature of the problem of child abuse; the finding of major blunt abdominal trauma should arouse a high index of suspicion. In addition to blunt abdominal trauma, children frequently have immersion or scald burns. The computed tomography scan should play a significant role in the screening of patients with this suspected diagnosis and abdominal findings.*

The Acute Abdomen in the Immunocompromised Host

Nylander WA Jr
Surg Clin North Am 68:457–469, April 1988 **5–26**

Some causes of acute abdomen are closely allied to a state of immune compromise. Active cytomegalovirus infection in the abdomen is diagnosed by tissue biopsy. Neutropenic enterocolitis is the most common form of acute abdomen in acute leukemics. Hepatitis can be caused by cytomegalovirus or Epstein-Barr virus infection. Hepatosplenic fungal microabscesses may produce an acute abdomen in an immunosuppressed patient. Small bowel perforation is a complication of lymphoma. Acute graft-versus-host disease may appear as acute abdomen. Perforation of the colon formerly was common after renal transplantation. Acute appendicitis is rare in immunosuppressed hosts apart from children receiving chemotherapy for leukemia. In all instances, the "pseudoacute abdomen," caused by colonic distention, must be kept in mind.

▶ *Acute abdomen in these patients poses several problems. In addition to the specific lesions noted in this article, it must be appreciated that patients who are immunocompromised may respond in a different fashion, and all of the classic signs and manifestations of perforation or ischemia may not pertain. If an acute surgical abdomen is in question, early exploration is indicated rather than waiting for the evolution of physical findings that verify the diagnosis.*

Bypass Surgery for Unresectable Oesophageal Cancer: Early and Late Results in 124 Cases

Mannell A, Becker PJ, Nissenbaum M
Br J Surg 75:283–286, March 1988 **5–27**

Most of a series of 124 patients with unresectable esophageal cancer had tumors 10 cm or less in length that invaded the mediastinum, but one fourth had more extensive tumors and, sometimes, fixed lymph nodes. In nearly all patients the entire stomach was used for bypass. Irradiation was a planned part of management. Operative mortality was 4%, and overall median survival was 5 months. Importantly, 90% of survivors were able to take an unrestricted diet and nearly as many gained weight.

▶ *This is a truly extraordinary experience when you look at the numbers of patients, the low operative mortality, and the percentage of survivors who had lasting relief from dysphagia. Wong and associates (*World J Surg *5:547, 1981) reported on 142 patients with unresectable tumors of the esophagus who underwent the Kirshner operation for palliation. In this procedure the esophageal obstruction was bypassed by subcutaneous or retrosternal gastric esophagoplasty, and the thoracic esophagus was defunctionalized by a long Roux-en-Y loop to the abdominal esophagus. The mortality in Wong's patients was almost 42%; the ability to eat normally was restored in 69% of survivors, and 28% were able to tolerate a soft diet.*

Prospective Controlled Vagotomy Trial for Duodenal Ulcer: Results After 11–15 Years

Hoffmann J, Jensen H-E, Christiansen J, et al
Ann Surg 209:40–45, January 1989 **5–28**

It still is necessary to ask what the best technique of vagotomy is for duodenal ulcer, and a definitive answer remains elusive. A series of 250 patients had elective surgery by 1 of 3 methods: either truncal or selective vagotomy combined with a drainage procedure, or parietal cell vagotomy. Ulcer disease recurred in 30% to 40% of patients in each group. Severe dumping was less of a risk after parietal cell vagotomy than after selective vagotomy. Dyspepsia was least frequent with parietal cell vagotomy, whereas diarrhea was infrequent in all groups. Perhaps two thirds of the patients overall ultimately were satisfied with the outcome, but sometimes only after prolonged medical care or a second operation. It may be time to consider vagotomy and antrectomy, even though postgastrectomy symptoms may be a frequent problem.

▶ *The incidence of peptic ulcer has decreased during the past decade, but interest in surgical management continues. Several articles have suggested that selective vagotomy and antrectomy remains the gold standard because it results in the smallest recurrence rate, but it causes the highest incidence of postvagotomy symptoms. Almost all trials agree that parietal cell vagotomy is associated with the lowest rate of severe postvagotomy symptoms. When managing an ulcer patient we have to weigh the risk of recurrence against that of the postvagotomy complications and then decide on the appropriate operation. For intractable ulcer pain, parietal cell vagotomy to me is currently the most attractive approach.*

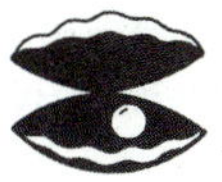

How long does the patient actually sit in the doctor's waiting room? An AMA survey showed an average of about 18 minutes. The shortest average waiting times were in the New England states (13:48) and the longest in the South (23:12).

Proximal Gastric Vagotomy: The Preferred Operation for Perforations in Acute Duodenal Ulcer

Boey J, Branicki FJ, Alagaratnam TT, et al
Ann Surg 208:169–174, August 1988 **5–29**

Symptomatic relapse is frequent when acute perforated duodenal ulcers are simply closed. Seventy-eight patients were assigned to have either closure alone or closure with proximal gastric vagotomy. After 3 years, more than a third of the patients undergoing simple closure had recurrences, and half of them required reoperation. Only 10% of the vagotomy group had recurrences. Proximal gastric vagotomy did not lead to dumping, diarrhea, or other serious side effects. The benefits of immediate proximal gastric vagotomy can be extended safely to many patients with acute perforation.

▶ *In most centers perforated peptic ulcers are managed by plication without a definitive antiacid drug procedure. Throughout the years there has been recurring interest in coupling the plication with a definitive procedure. Proximal gastric vagotomy is the ideal approach because it is not associated with the complications of dumping, diarrhea, and other side effects associated with truncal vagotomy and drainage procedures or with truncal vagotomy and antrectomy. Given the low risk of this procedure coupled with the recurrence rates reported in this article, the authors make a strong case that this is the initial procedure of choice.*

Current Status of Proximal Gastric Vagotomy

Schirmer BD
Ann Surg 209:131–148, February 1989 **5–30**

Proximal gastric vagotomy has been around for nearly 2 decades and has been scrutinized more closely than any other ulcer operation. The conclusion: When performed by an experienced surgeon, it is the preferred approach to chronic duodenal ulcer after medical treatment has failed. The operation counters gastric acid production without altering motility substantially. The low rate of side effects is a very appealing aspect of proximal vagotomy; a relatively high rate of recurrent ulcer is its chief drawback. The role of proximal gastric vagotomy in treating complications of peptic ulcer disease remains cloudy.

▶ *This is an up-to-date status report about a procedure truly regarded as the treatment of choice for chronic duodenal ulcer for patients in whom other therapy has failed. The recurrence rate, although admittedly greater than with truncal vagotomy and antrectomy, is reasonable, but the satisfaction index is significantly higher than that associated with the latter procedure. Some of the advocates of proximal vagotomy use it in association with dilation of the pylorus or to relieve obstruction, combining it with ligation of bleeding vessels at the base of the ulcer, but most reserve the operation for patients with retractable pain. In those patients without significant soilage of the peritoneal cavity, it is reasonable to treat perforation by plication and proximal gastric vagotomy.*

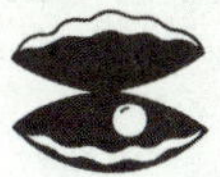

The AMA Socioeconomic Monitoring System reports that the average physician sees about 120 patients per week. The number has been dropping steadily since the early 1980s.

Mesenteric Ischemia

Williams LF Jr
Surg Clin North Am 68:331–353, April 1988 **5–31**

An early and precise diagnosis of extensive mesenteric ischemia is critical. The chief possibilities are arterial embolism or thrombus, venous occlusion, and nonocclusive ischemia caused by low blood flow. The initial test is flush aortography with selective injections. The Doppler method and fluorescein dye injection now make it easier to assess bowel viability at laparotomy. Vasodilators are an important adjunct to resection. Chronic mucosal infarction of long segments of small bowel can follow successful treatment of acute extensive mesenteric ischemia. Limited mesenteric ischemia is most often caused by ischemic colitis.

▶ *As the mean age of the population increases, mesenteric ischemia is becoming a more frequent entity. The best prognosis remains in patients with limited ischemic segments, usually related to venous thrombosis. Although we would anticipate that mesenteric ischemia related to arterial embolism would have a more favorable prognosis, such has not been the case in most studies. The poor prognosis associated with nonocclusive ischemia caused by low blood flow relates to the basic disease that causes the low-flow state.*

Ulcerative Colitis and Polyposis Coli: Surgical Options

Sackier JM, Wood CB
Surg Clin North Am 68:1319–1338, December 1988 **5–32**

Pouch surgery for ulcerative colitis and polyposis coli aims at both cure and continence. Various pouch types are available. In the modified S design, 2 of 3 15-cm limbs are opened and anastomosed. In the J pouch, the distal ileum is turned back on itself, and the apex is anastomosed to the anus (Fig 5–1). The new perimuscular rectal dissection technique minimizes bladder and bowel dysfunction. The Coloshield intraluminal bypass tube protects anastomoses by diverting fecal flow away from the suture or staple lines. After surgery, use of a rectal probe stimulator can lessen fecal incontinence.

▶ *One of the most important advances in intestinal surgery in the past decade has been the application of so-called pouch procedures to provide both cure and continence for patients with ulcerative colitis*

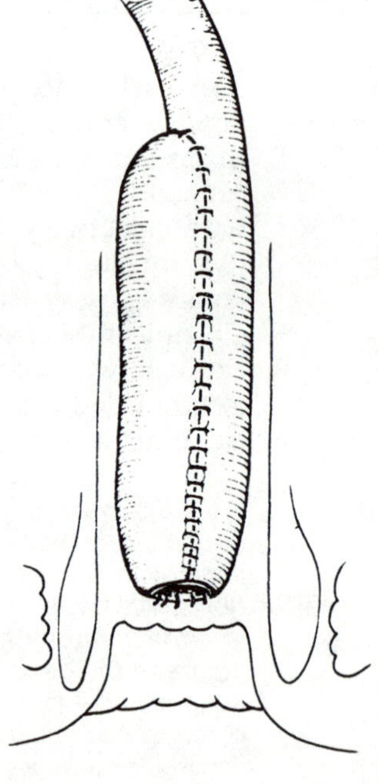

Fig 5–1
The J pouch as proposed by Utsonomiya showing the 2 limbs and the pouch-anal anastomosis. (Courtesy of Sackier JM, Wood CB: *Surg Clin North Am* 68:1319–1338, December 1988.)

and polyposis coli. In the past it was believed that an intact rectal mucosa was required to establish a reflex arc that would insure continence. Only after it was realized that rectal mucosa was not required to maintain continence and that the sole requirement was sympathetic and parasympathetic innovation of the levators and sphincters did this surgical approach evolve. The pouch procedure is not applicable in patients with Crohn's colitis, and an alternative procedure for management of polyposis coli is still ileoproctostomy with surveillance of the residual rectal mucosa.

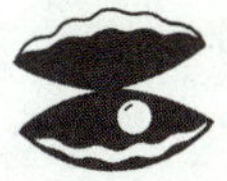

If you tell your patients to exercise, what are they likely to do? About 68 million Americans bowl, 41 million play softball, 22 million golf, and 17 million swing tennis rackets.

Conservative Treatment of Distal Rectal Cancer by Local Excision

DeCosse JJ, Wong RJ, Quan SHQ, et al
Cancer 63:219–223, Jan 15, 1989 **5–33**

Perhaps half of all large bowel cancers are localized at the time of diagnosis and therefore are amenable to local excision. In a series of 57 patients who had full-thickness excision of distal rectal cancer, 10% died specifically of the disease. Of 27 patients lacking adverse risk factors such as a mucin-producing tumor or full-thickness invasion, none died. Ulceration or involvement of the muscularis alone did not compromise the outcome. Adjuvant radiotherapy may confer some protection, and abdominal perineal resection may be done if cancer recurs locally.

▶ *All aspects of modern surgery are being permeated with attempts to be more conservative about extirpation of malignant tumors. This article represents yet another sample. Selection is the essence for application of the principle of surgical treatment for distal rectal cancer, particularly for lesions that show evidence of penetration. The fact that mucinous characteristics and full-thickness invasion are associated with an adverse outcome aids in determining the applicability of this approach to a given patient.*

Sphincter-Saving Procedures for Distal Carcinoma of the Rectum

Yeatman TJ, Bland KI
Ann Surg 209:1–18, January 1989 **5–34**

A sphincter-saving operation has been developed for use at every level of the rectum, and abdominoperineal resection is done less often today. Significant extra rectal length can be gained if the rectum is properly dissected circumferentially to the levator ani (Fig 5–2). Generally, adequate functional results are obtained from a wide range of restorative operations. No matter what technique is used, pelvic recurrences are a problem in patients with low-lying cancers.

► *The sphincter-saving procedure described here began because of the demonstration that fecal continence is derived from the mechanical action of the anal sphincters innovated by sympathetic and parasympathetic fibers and* not *dependent on an intact rectum. The authors are certainly justified in the prediction that permanent abdominal colostomy and abdominoperineal resection may become increasingly rare.*

Preoperative Irradiation for Rectal Cancer: Improved Local Control and Long-Term Survival

Kodner IJ, Shemesh EI, Fry RD, et al
Ann Surg 209:194–199, February 1989 **5–35**

Does it help to irradiate rectal cancer patients before excisional surgery? Doses of 2,000 and 4,500 cGY were tested in more than 100 patients having transmurally invasive adenocarcinoma. With both doses the 5-year survival was about 85%, and fewer than 2% of patients had local recurrence. Radiotherapy definitely makes these tumors more resectable. These results, however, did not include patients having fixed, poorly differentiated tumors. Efforts now are needed to control colorectal cancer systemically.

► *The survival rates achieved in this series are the best that have been reported, and the local recurrence rates are also the best reported to date. It must be pointed out, however, that studies from other institutions have demonstrated that although preoperative radiation of the pelvis reduced local recurrence, it did not affect the survival rates.*

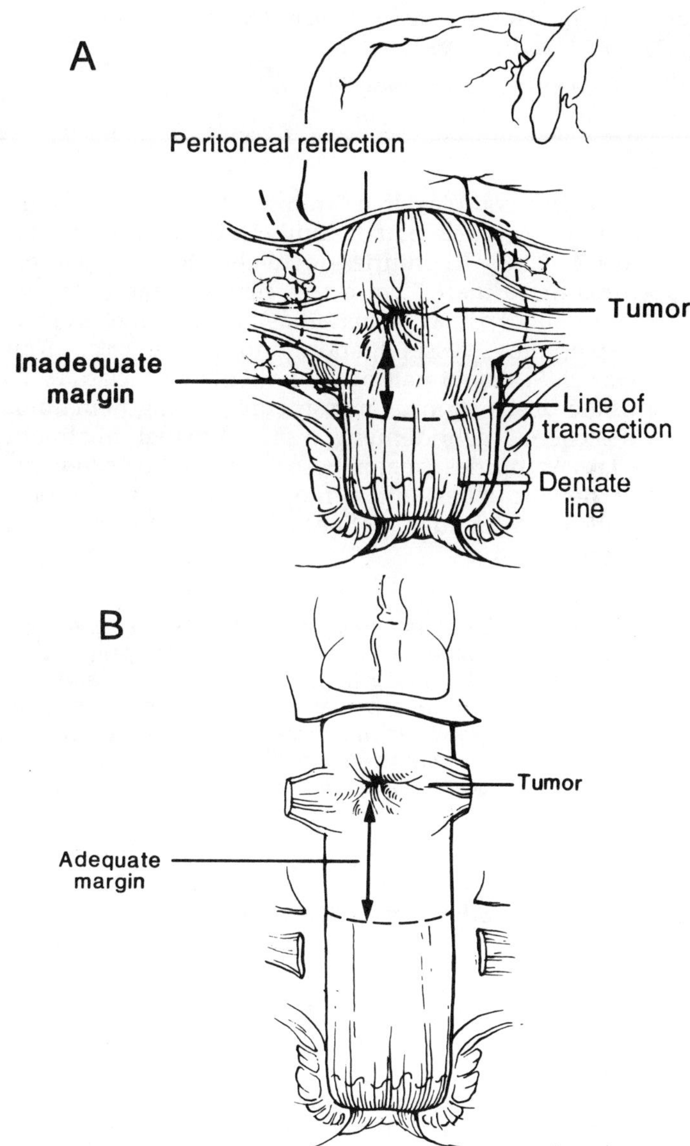

Fig 5–2
Abdominal dissection may serve to lengthen distal tumor-free margins and permit sphincter preservation. **A,** before dissection, margin inadequate. **B,** after dissection, margin adequate. (Courtesy of Yeatman TJ, Bland KI: *Ann Surg* 209:1–18, January 1989.)

Severe Hepatic Trauma: A Multi-Center Experience With 1,335 Liver Injuries

Cogbill TH, Moore EE, Jurkovich GJ, et al
J Trauma 28:1433–1438, October 1988 **5–36**

The 210 complex liver injuries treated at 6 regional trauma centers included equal numbers of penetrating and blunt injuries. Class III injuries (actively bleeding parenchymal fractures more than 3 cm deep, central penetrating wounds, and large subcapsular hematomas) most often were managed by hepatotomy, vessel ligation, and deep liver suturing. Mortality was 25%. About half of the patients with class IV lesions (lobar tissue destruction or massive expanding hematoma) survived; resectional débridement was the usual treatment approach. Class V injuries (major vessel damage or extensive disruption of hepatic lobes) often required caval shunt placement, but only 4 of 59 such patients lived; earlier shunting might be more effective.

► *Management of major injuries to the liver remains a significant challenge. These authors emphasize the high mortality in patients with retrohepatic caval or major hepatic venous injuries and the low yield associated with the caval catheter. The use of packs as a temporary tamponade to be removed in several days is now accepted as a valuable adjunct in the management of these patients. Because of the large number of patients evaluated in this report, the data are most meaningful.*

Preoperative Chemotherapy in "Unresectable" Hepatoblastoma

Pierro A, Langevin AM, Filler RM, et al
J Pediatr Surg 24:24–29, January 1989 **5–37**

Eleven children with "unresectable" hepatoblastomas—8 with hepatoblastoma in both lobes of the liver and 3 others with very large tumors—received preoperative chemotherapy. This included doxorubicin hydrochloride (Adriamycin) for all patients and cisplatin for most of them. After 2–6 cycles of treatment, 8 tumors were less than half as extensive as at the outset, and metastases disappeared in 2 patients. Attempts at removing disease completely succeeded in 7 of 8 patients, and these children were doing well at follow-up 4–42 months later. Two children with anaplastic tumors died.

▶ *The demonstration that chemotherapy can alter the resectability of a hepatoblastoma and that cures can be effected in these patients is extremely important. The response reported is unique for hepatoblastoma, but unfortunately does not pertain to hepatocellular carcinomas. The question of whether chemotherapy should be applied to all patients has been raised, but because of the drug toxicity this is not generally applied.*

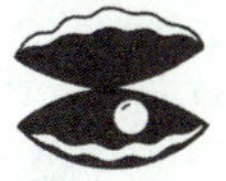

Leonardo Da Vinci is said to have recognized the first case of congenital heart disease: an atrial septal defect in 1531.

Personal Experience With 411 Hepatic Resections

Iwatsuki S, Starzl TE
Ann Surg 208:421–434, October 1988 **5–38**

The number of partial hepatic resections performed each year continues to increase. About one fourth of resections performed at 2 sites in 2 decades were for primary liver tumor, and another fourth were for hepatic metastases, most often from colorectal cancer. Resections ranged from local excision to trisegmentectomy and lobectomy. Operative mortality was 3%, and 6 additional late deaths resulted from resectional liver failure. Bile leakage tended to occur after left trisegmentectomy. When patients with benign disease survived hepatic resection, the risk of the original disease recurring was minimal, and no liability from the resection itself was noted. Although liver resection now is relatively safe, a nonoperative approach to malignant disease will prove best.

▶ *This article brings into focus the low risk that is now associated with major hepatic resection. Although certain caveats pertain, hepatic resection is rarely indicated for focal nodular hyperplasia and more than 90% of hemangiomas can be managed nonoperatively. The question of extensive hepatic resection in the face of cirrhosis is not resolved by this paper.*

Resection of the Liver for Colorectal Carcinoma Metastases: A Multi-Institutional Study of Indications for Resection

Registry of Hepatic Metastases
Surgery 103:278–288, March 1988 **5–39**

After 5 years, more than 800 patients from 24 centers who had liver resection for metastatic colorectal cancer, one third survived, and one fifth survived without disease. Possible contraindications to this surgery are positive hepatic nodes, resectable extrahepatic metastases, and 4 or more metastases. The resection margins and the disease-free interval also should be considered before recommending resection. Anatomical resection often is less complicated than a large wedge resection and causes less blood loss; it is the best approach when metastases larger than 4 cm are present.

▶ *This article adds reinforcement to the thesis that resection of the liver for colorectal carcinoma in selected patients results in a higher survival rate than resection of primary tumors in other gastrointestinal organs such as the esophagus, the stomach, and pancreas. The data did not resolve the issue of resection for bilobular disease. The 2 5-year survivors might still have lived if resection had not been performed. More data certainly are required to address this issue. We must remind ourselves not to compare our achievements with the figures put forth by Jaffe et al. (*Surg Gynecol Obstet *127:1, 1968) because we see a different subset of patients with metastatic disease, those detected by imaging techniques, and many of our resections are performed in patients with large solitary lesions. The natural history of these biologic lesions has not been defined.*

The Role of Liver Transplantation in Hepatobiliary Malignancy: A Retrospective Analysis of 95 Patients With Particular Regard to Tumor Stage and Recurrence

Ringe B, Wittekind C, Bechstein WO, et al
Ann Surg 209:88–98, January 1989 **5–40**

Does liver transplantation have a place in the management of unresectable liver or bile duct cancer? Malignancy, most often hepatocellular and bile duct carcinoma, accounted for one third of liver transplants in a 15-year series. Nine patients with liver

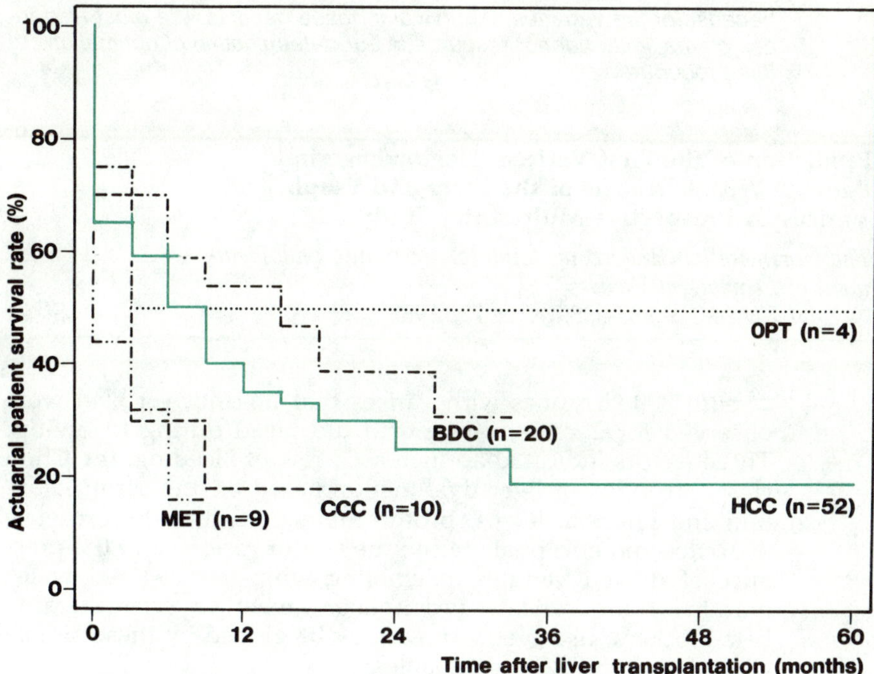

Fig 5–3
Results of liver transplantation according to the histologic type of tumor. *Abbreviations: HCC,* hepatocellular carcinoma; *CCC,* cholangiocellular carcinoma; *OPT,* other primary liver tumors; *BDC,* bile duct carcinoma; *MET,* liver metastases. (Courtesy of Ringe B, Wittekind C, Bechstein WO, et al: *Ann Surg* 209:88–98, January 1989.)

metastasis were included. The survival rate at 5 years was 20%, but the median survival has risen substantially in the past few years. Patients with disease limited to the liver had the best outcome; those with hepatocellular cancer had a median survival of 10 years (Fig 5–3). The bad news is that patients with liver metastasis or cholangiocellular cancer did not live long. Hepatobiliary cancer does not preclude liver transplantation, but careful patient selection is critical. Adjuvant chemotherapy and immunotherapy may help save even more of these patients in the future.

▶ *This is one of the more encouraging reports on the subject. Most series have not had equivalently good results; the results with proximal bile duct cancer have been particularly poor. As the authors point out, the contribution of transplantation to long-term cure is hard to assess because of the vagaries of survival in these patients. We must also focus on the limited donor resource in our determination of optimal use of this procedure.*

Prediction of the First Variceal Hemorrhage in Patients With Cirrhosis of the Liver and Esophageal Varices: A Prospective Multicenter Study

The North Italian Endoscopic Club for the Study and Treatment of Esophageal Varices
N Engl J Med 319:983–989, Oct 13, 1988 **5–41**

About 300 cirrhotics with varices that had not yet bled were observed for 2 years; one fourth did bleed during follow-up. Three factors indicated an increased risk of bleeding: the Child class, an index of liver dysfunction based on the serum albumin and bilirubin levels, prothrombin time, and the presence of ascites and encephalopathy; the size of varices; and the presence of dilated venules resembling whip marks ("red wale" markings) on varices. Prophylaxis, whether sclerotherapy, beta-blockers, or surgery, now may be guided by these simple clinical and endoscopic variables.

▶ *This article allows us to focus on a group of patients for whom a prophylactic shunting procedure may be appropriate. As the authors point out, all major trials so far have indicated that a prophylactic portacaval shunt fails to prolong survival. We used to believe that it was impossible to identify patients who were likely to bleed. The next step is to recognize the patients with a predictably high incidence of bleeding and subject them to a variety of prophylactic therapeutic regimens, including sclerotherapy, devascularization procedures, and shunts.*

A Retrospective Analysis of 3 Years' Experience of an Interdisciplinary Approach to Gallstone Disease Including Shock-Waves

Heberer G, Paumgartner G, Sauerbruch T, et al
Ann Surg 208:274–278, September 1988 **5–42**

One fourth of 1,200 patients with gallstone disease underwent extracorporeal shock-wave lithotripsy with no deaths. With shock-wave treatment and medical dissolution, 90% of patients were free of stones after 2 years. Operative mortality of patients undergoing elective operation was less than 1%. Complications occurred in 4% of patients who had the operation and in 7% of those given shock-wave therapy. Three fourths of patients with bile duct stones had endoscopic sphincterotomy with lithotripsy added if necessary; 3 patients required reoperation for retained fragments. This is the preferred approach to bile duct stones, but surgery will remain the dominant treatment for gallstone disease for at least the next decade.

▶ *This represents the most definitive work in the field. The use of lithotripsy for biliary calculi is increasing geometrically. However, several major issues need to be defined by cooperative studies: (1) The subset of patients to be treated will have to be precisely defined. It must be appreciated that the circumstance is quite dissimilar from ureteral calculi, where one is not dealing with the diseased organ. On the occasion of the first paper describing elective cholecystectomy, Langenbush wrote, "The gallbladder is removed not because it contains stones but because it forms stones." This implies that a diseased organ will be left in place and symptoms may be related to the organ rather than to the stones themselves. At this point, it is anticipated that only about 15% of patients considered for gallstone lithotripsy will meet the therapeutic requirements, and adjunctive dissolution therapy is necessary. At this point, cholecystectomy remains the treatment of choice for most patients with symptomatic gallstones.*

Acute Cholecystitis in the Diabetic: A Case-Control Study of Outcome

Hickman MS, Schwesinger WH, Page CP
Arch Surg 123:409–411, April 1988 **5–43**

Should diabetics with asymptomatic gallstones have prophylactic cholecystectomy? In a controlled study of 72 diabetics requiring urgent surgery, pathology was not more marked than in controls, but morbidity was nearly twice as frequent in diabetics. Infectious complications were threefold more frequent, and all 3 patients who died were diabetics with sepsis. The issue of what to do with asymptomatic patients remains open, but, without question, diabetics with symptomatic gallstones require expeditious operation.

▶ *The findings of this study suggest that diabetic patients with cholelithiasis should undergo elective operation to obviate the complications associated with the development of acute cholecystitis. At present, no data actually settle the controversy of the role of prophylactic cholecystectomy in asymptomatic diabetic patients. Data indicating the number of diabetic patients with cholelithiasis who will ultimately experience the acute complications of biliary tract disease are required.*

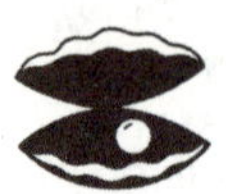

Willem Einthoven of The Netherlands won the Nobel prize in 1924 for developing a device for recording the electrical activity of the heart. The first device, manufactured in Germany, was called an *elektrokardiogramm,* thus the common abbreviation, EKG. *ECG,* reflecting the English spelling, is now in more common use.

Gallstone Pancreatitis: A Prospective Randomized Trial of the Timing of Surgery

Kelly TR, Wagner DS
Surgery 104:600–605, October 1988 **5–44**

Is it better to operate right away on gallstone pancreatitis or to wait 48 hours? The message from a series of 165 patients is, first, in patients with mild pancreatitis the timing of surgery makes little difference. Second, in patients with severe pancreatitis early surgery worsens the outcome. Apparently, gallstones initiate pancreatitis, but its course depends on the amount of digestive enzymes activated, not on the stones themselves. Surgery is best deferred until pancreatitis has subsided.

▶ *Mercer et al.* (Am J Surg *148:749, 1984) reviewed the results of operation in 34 patients with gallstone pancreatitis and found that operation was the preferred treatment. Frei et al.* (Am J Surg *151:170, 1986) reviewed 153 patients who underwent cholecystectomy for treatment of biliary pancreatitis. Conservative management with scheduled readmission was associated with a highly unacceptable recurrence rate of biliary pancreatitis, leading those authors to agree that early operations are indicated.*

Chronic Pancreatitis: Results of Whipple's Resection and Total Pancreatectomy

Stone WM, Sarr MG, Nagorney DM, et al
Arch Surg 123:815–819, July 1988 **5–45**

Fifteen patients with chronic pancreatitis underwent partial pancreatoduodenectomy (Whipple's resection), and an equal number had total gland resection. Three patients in each group had major morbidity, but there were no operative deaths. Twelve patients had significant relief of pain after a Whipple resection, and 10 had relief after total pancreatectomy. In neither group was the outcome predicted by the cause of pancreatitis, the presence of gland calcification, or even abstinence from alcohol. If the pancreatic duct is dilated, a duct drainage procedure probably is best, preserving pancreatic substance. If, however, patients experience incapacitating pain and no substantial duct dilation, resection can be planned. The type of resection depends on the extent and primary site of disease as well as on endocrine and exocrine function.

▶ *The indication for operative intervention in patients with chronic pancreatitis is intractable pain. The failure to alleviate pain by removing most or all of the pancreas is disappointing and probably relates in part to the drug dependency of many of these patients. Total pancreatectomy in patients with labile diabetes should be avoided in those who are drug dependent because they are frequently noncompliant about their insulin therapy and deaths have occurred because of hyperglycemia or, more often, hypoglycemia.*

Total Pancreatectomy for Ductal Adenocarcinoma of the Pancreas: An Update

van Heerdan JA, McIlrath DC, Ilstrup DM, et al
World J Surg 12:658–662, October 1988 **5–46**

From 1951 to 1985, 90 patients with ductal adenocarcinoma, half of them with positive peripancreatic nodes, underwent total pancreatectomy. The operative mortality final survival rate was about 10%, and the median survival time was 1 year. As with other measures, initial optimism about total pancreatectomy has waned. True, the operative risk has been reduced in recent years, but no substantial improvement in long-term survival has resulted. This surgery is warranted only if radical pancreatoduodenectomy is not feasible.

▶ *The 3- and 5-year survival rates of 11% and 7%, respectively, are in keeping with most reports. The authors demonstrate that total pancreatectomy adds little to classic pancreaticoduodenectomy in terms of decreasing hospital mortality or improving long-term survival. A report from the Gastrointestinal Tumor Study Group and the Johns Hopkins Hospital indicates that the 5-year survival rate in patients with uninvolved nodes may be as high as 40%. In adjudicating these disparate findings, I point out that most centers believe a 5-year cure of carcinoma of the pancreas is an anecdotal experience.*

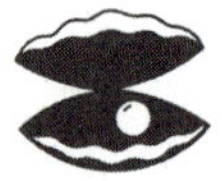

According to the 1988 U.S. Census Bureau report, the average daily hospital room rate was $253. The highest average was in Washington, D.C. ($443), the lowest in Mississippi ($141).

Splenic Injury: A 5-Year Update With Improved Results and Changing Criteria for Conservative Management

Pearl RH, Wesson DE, Spence LJ, et al
J Pediatr Surg 24:121–125, January 1989 **5–47**

Of 75 children with splenic injury, caused most often by car accidents, 10 required surgery, 7 of whom lived. All of the 65 patients managed without operation survived. Only 1 of 45 patients with injury of the spleen alone required laparotomy. Only 15 patients treated without operation received transfusions. Of the conservatively treated patients, 20 received intensive care for 3 days on average. None had delayed splenic ruptures. Selective nonoperative management avoids such complications as bowel obstruction and abscess formation as well as the risk of postsplenectomy sepsis.

▶ *The policy of conservative nonoperative management of the injured spleen is a concept of our decade. The overwhelming majority of patients in the pediatric age group can be managed conservatively. An appreciable but smaller percentage of adults can be managed in a similar fashion. If, however, a question of multiple organ involvement arises, or if massive hemorrhage has occurred, splenectomy should not be delayed.*

Splenectomy for Immune Thrombocytopenia Related to Human Immunodeficiency Virus

Ferguson CM
Surg Gynecol Obstet 167:300–302, October 1988 **5–48**

Thrombocytopenia associated with HIV infection resembles classic immune thrombocytopenic purpura clinically, although a specific platelet antigen is responsible. Eleven patients had their spleens removed for this reason, 6 after a trial of steroids. All of the patients had an immediate and excellent response to splenectomy with no important complications. Splenectomy is a safe, effective initial treatment for HIV-infected patients with immune thrombocytopenic purpura.

▶ *As we would expect, the results in this subset of patients are similar to the results in those patients affected with idiopathic thrombocytopenic purpura. A platelet rise to 100,000/mm^3 is expected in 85% of patients with idiopathic thrombocytopenic purpura after splenectomy; in the 15% of patients whose counts do not achieve this level, ecchymosis and purpura rarely occur subsequent to splenectomy. The finding that lack of response to steroids does not militate against a favorable response to splenectomy is in keeping with the experience of patients with idiopathic thrombocytopenic purpura.*

Indications and Results for Splenectomy for Beta Thalassemia in Two Hundred and Twenty-One Pediatric Patients

Pinna AD, Argiolu F, Marongiu L, et al
Surg Gynecol Obstet 167:109–113, August 1988 **5–49**

The outcome of splenectomy was compared in 221 children with β-thalassemia and 61 children with other disorders. Complications were far more frequent in thalassemic patients. Of 7 deaths, 6 resulted from overwhelming postsplenectomy infection. The good news is that blood consumption declined by nearly half, and hemoglobin levels rose substantially in survivors. Splenectomy does improve the quality of life in children with β-thalassemia and reduces medical costs. The use of platelet antiaggregant and antibiotic drugs after surgery will make thrombotic and septic problems less likely to occur.

▶ *This is the largest reported series where splenectomy was carried out for an uncommon congenital hemolytic anemia. We should emphasize that the high incidence of infection in these patients was augmented by the removal of the spleen. However, there is little question that splenectomy for β-thalassemia improves the quality of life of many patients. Antibiotic prophylaxis probably should be maintained throughout life in these patients. The incidence of overwhelming postsplenectomy infection in patients with hereditary spherocytosis is significantly less, and it is probably reasonable to maintain antibiotics in patients with spherocytosis until age 18 years.*

Experience With Simultaneous Pancreas-Kidney Transplantation

Sollinger HW, Stratta RJ, D'Alessandro AM, et al
Ann Surg 208:475–483, October 1988 **5–50**

Transplantation of the vascularized pancreas now is a practical possibility. A group of 30 patients who had juvenile-onset diabetes for 2 decades received a pancreatic transplant with pancreatico-duodenocystostomy at the same time as renal transplantation. All patients were immediately independent of insulin. Most patients had more than 1 rejection episode, but 94% of kidneys and 84% of the pancreas grafts survived at 2 years. The mean serum creatinine level was 1.75 mg/dL at time of publication. The 1 death resulted from rupture of a mycotic aneurysm at the site of the pancreatic arterial anastomosis. In selected juvenile diabetics, transplantation of a pancreas and a kidney from the same donor will lessen neuropathy and microvascular disease and improve the quality of life.

▶ *As the discussants of this paper point out, it is paradoxical that the transplant success rate is higher when kidney and pancreas are transplanted simultaneously than when pancreas transplantation is performed either before or after kidney transplantation. It remains to be shown whether pancreatic transplantation does anything other than obviate the need for exogenous insulin. Early studies have indicated that retinopathy does not change after pancreas transplant.*

Cadaveric Renal Transplantation in the Cyclosporine and OKT_3 Eras

Stratta RJ, D'Alessandro AM, Hoffmann RM, et al
Surgery 104:606–615, October 1988 **5–51**

All 500 patients receiving cadaver kidney grafts were treated with prednisone, azathioprine, antilymphoblast globulin, and cyclosporine. About half of these patients were eligible to receive the monoclonal antibody OKT3 for resistant rejection. The actuarial patient survival rate was 90% at 3 years. About 80% of primary renal grafts and 60% of nonprimary grafts survived. In the OKT3 era patient survival has improved to 98% and primary graft survival at 1 year has reached 91%. Almost two thirds of 49 grafts were rescued after OKT3 treatment. Results in insulin-dependent diabetics have improved. Prospective tissue matching and prophylaxis with OKT3 may bring even better results to high-risk patients.

▸ *This is the current state-of-the-art. Other investigators have noted that primary graft nonfunction is reduced from about 7% to 2% when the administration of cyclosporine is delayed. Review of the world's literature suggests that this 4-drug immunosuppressive regimen for kidney transplantation is associated with the best results.*

The Undescended Testis: Hormonal and Surgical Management

Elder JS
Surg Clin North Am 68:983–1005, October 1988 **5–52**

In patients with cryptorchidism, the most common disorder of male sexual differentiation, the physician should determine whether the testis has been felt in the scrotum previously and should inquire into urinary problems. Complications of an undescended testis include both infertility and testicular cancer. Chorionic gonadotropin is used to stimulate the normal androgen-mediated process of testicular descent. A gonadotropin-releasing hormone analogue may be able to stimulate germ cell development in the cryptorchid testis. Laparoscopy is being used increasingly to localize the impalpable testis, which can generally be fixed in the scrotum as an outpatient procedure (orchiopexy). A gel-filled testicular prosthesis now is available for use when a testis is missing.

▶ *The management of this common disorder is critical, although orchiopexy does not appear to lessen the risk of testicular cancer. The relative ineffectiveness of human chorionic gonadotropin or gonadotropin-releasing hormone emphasizes the need for orchiopexy.*

ANNOTATED BIBLIOGRAPHY

INTERNAL MEDICINE

Blumberg BS, Alter HJ, Visnich S: A "new" antigen in leukemia sera. *JAMA* 191:541–546, 1965.

▸ This article delineates the discovery of hepatitis B virus.

Brown MS, Goldstein JL: Expression of the familial hypercholesterolemia gene in heterozygotes: Mechanism for a dominant disorder in man. *Science* 185:61–63, 1974.

▸ The paper that eventually led to a Nobel Prize, showing a specific low-density lipoprotein receptor defect.

Dicken CH: Retinoids: A review. *J Am Acad Dermatol* 11:541–552, 1984.

▸ Retinoids, synthetic derivatives of vitamin A, have assumed an important role in the treatment of many skin diseases, particularly acne and a number of disorders of keratinization.

Gottlieb MS, Schroff R, Schanker HM, et al: *Pneumocystis carinii* pneumonia and mucosal candidiasis in previously healthy homosexual men. *N Engl J Med* 305:1425–1431, 1981.

▸ First description of the clinical complex that we now recognize as acquired immunodeficiency syndrome, i.e., AIDS.

Gregory RA, Tracy HJ: The constitution and properties of two gastrins extracted from hog antral mucosa. I. The isolation of two gastrins from hog antral mucosa. II. The properties of two gastrins isolated from hog antral mucosa. *Gut* 5:103–117, 1964.

▸ These landmark papers describe the characteristics of gastrin.

Koch-Weser J: The serum level approach to individualization of drug dosage. *Eur J Clin Pharmacol* 9:1–8, 1975.

▸ A classic relating to monitoring of drug levels.

Petty TL, Stanford RE, Neff TA: Continuous oxygen therapy in chronic airway obstruction. *Ann Intern Med* 75:361–367, 1971.

▸ This article was the first to show that continuous oxygen therapy increases patient survival.

Plum F, Posner JB: *The Diagnosis of Stupor and Coma.* Philadelphia, FA Davis Co, 1980.

▶ This emphasizes bedside evaluation and clinical neuroanatomical correlations, and provides a conceptual framework for dealing with unexplained stupor or coma.

Posternak L, Brunner HR, Gavras H, et al: Angiotensin II blockade in normal man: Interaction of renin and sodium in maintaining blood pressure. *Kidney Int* 11:197–203, 1977.

▶ Normal individuals, on a low Na diet, use the renin-angiotensin system to maintain normal blood pressure.

Shapiro S: Evidence on screening for breast cancer from a randomized trial. *Cancer* 39:2772–2782, 1977.

▶ This is the major report of the results of the "HIP" study (Health Insurance Plan of Greater New York), which first demonstrated that screening mammography can reduce mortality from breast cancer.

OBSTETRICS AND GYNECOLOGY

Fisk NM: Modifications to selective conservative management in preterm premature rupture of the membranes. *Obstet Gynecol Surv* 43:328–334, June 1988.

▸ This article is an excellent review of conservative management of patients with preterm rupture of the membranes, an important aspect of the management of premature labor.

King CR: Prenatal diagnosis of genetic disease with molecular genetic technology. *Obstet Gynecol Surv* 43:493–508, September 1988.

▸ The ability to perform sophisticated genetic technology is thoroughly reviewed in this article.

Koss LG: The Papanicolaou test for cervical cancer detection: A triumph and a tragedy. *JAMA* 261:737–743, February 1989.

▸ The positives and negatives of Papanicolaou's smear for cervical cancer detection are thoroughly discussed in this review article.

Meehan FP: Delivery following prior cesarean section: An obstetrician's dilemma? *Obstet Gynecol Surv* 43:582–589, October 1988.

▸ Vaginal birth after cesarean section (VBAC) is now an accepted entity in the United States; this article reviews the pros and cons of VBAC.

Spielman FJ, Herbert WNP: Maternal cardiovascular effects of drugs that alter uterine activity. *Obstet Gynecol Surv* 43:516–522, September 1988.

▸ One of the exciting advances in recent times is the possibility that premature uterine activity can be suppppressed effectively; however, with this suppression come side effects, and this article is a good review of those associated with drugs altering uterine activity.

PEDIATRICS

Bart KJ, Hinman AR, Jordan WS, Jr: International Symposium on Vaccine Development and Utilization. *Rev Infect Dis* **11:S491–S667, 1989.**

▸ This international symposium on vaccine development details current up-to-date information with regard to presently licensed vaccines and those soon to be licensed, and provides detailed information on the efficacy rates, benefits, and potential risks of all available vaccines.

Campbell AGM: Immunization for the immunosuppressed child. *Arch Dis Child* **63:113–115, 1988.**

▸ This article details extremely important information about the response, or lack thereof, of the immunosuppressed child to various licensed vaccines. This information is not readily available from any other single source.

Falloon J, Eddy J, Wiener L, et al: Human immunodeficiency virus infection in children. *J Pediatr* **114:1–3, 1989.**

▸ This is a detailed, yet succinct, review of the present status of human immunodeficiency virus infection in children.

Johnson JP: Genetic counselling using linked DNA probes: Cystic fibrosis as a prototype. *J Pediatr* **113:957–967, 1988.**

▸ This review demonstrates the value of using linked DNA probes for the diagnosis of a large number of inherited diseases using cystic fibrosis (the most common inherited disease) as a prototype. It is an excellent review article for those who have a cursory knowledge of molecular biology and wish to learn more about this subject and its application to clinical problems.

Lin AN, Carter DM: Epidermolysis bullosa: When the skin falls apart. *J Pediatr* **114:349–355, 1989.**

▸ This is an excellent review of current information concerning epidermolysis bullosa, including its various clinical manifestations and modes of inheritance. The modern methods for establishing the diagnosis of each subtype definitively are detailed.

Osborne JP: Diagnosis of tuberous sclerosis. *Arch Dis Child* **63:1423–1425, 1988.**

▸ This is a succinct review of those clinical features that enable one to establish the diagnosis of tuberous sclerosis definitively.

Polkey CE: Surgery for epilepsy. *Arch Dis Child* **64:185–187, 1989.**

▸ This is a brief review of the appropriateness, or lack thereof, for surgery as a technique for the control of various seizure disorders of childhood.

Rosenberg AM: Advanced drug therapy for juvenile rheumatoid arthritis. *J Pediatr* 114:171–179, 1989.

▸ This excellent review covers the use of many licensed and soon to be licensed nonsteroidal anti-inflammatory agents for the treatment of juvenile rheumatoid arthritis. It contrasts their effectiveness with salicylate and steroid therapy.

Ware R: Human parvovirus infection. *J Pediatr* 114:343–349, 1989.

▸ This superb review details our current knowledge concerning the clinical diseases caused by parvoviruses.

Weinberg GA, Granoff DM: Polysaccharide-protein conjugate vaccines for the prevention of *Haemophilus influenzae,* type b disease. *J Pediatr* 113:621–631, 1988.

▸ This is a detailed review of the various polysaccharide-protein conjugate vaccines currently being tested to determine their efficacy in the prevention of *Hemophilus influenzae,* type b disease. These authors have simplified the presentation of a very complex field.

PSYCHIATRY

Feldman MD: The challenge of self-mutilation: A review. ***Compre Psychiatry*** **29:252–269, May–June 1988.**

▸ A comprehensive review of both the differing theories behind self-mutilation and the different treatment approaches.

Gerlach J, Casey DE: Tardive dyskinesia. ***Acta Psychiatr Scand*** **77:369–378, August 1988.**

▸ Although nothing new is revealed about this troubling side effect of neuroleptics, this review offers a nice summary of its clinical aspects, etiologic factors, prevention, and treatment approaches.

Harding JJ: Postpartum psychiatric disorders: A review. ***Compre Psychiatry*** **30:109–112, January–February 1989.**

▸ A good summary of what we know about "postpartum disorders," a category missing in *DSM-III-R* per se.

Scott J: Chronic depression. ***Br J Psychiatry*** **153:287–297, September 1988.**

▸ A very nice review of a frequent (12% to 15% prevalence), but infrequently written about, condition.

Stein D, Avni J: Thyroid hormones in the treatment of affective disorders. ***Acta Psychiatr Scand*** **77:623–636, December 1988.**

▸ This offers a good look at why thyroid, alone or with tricyclics, is used more and more often in the management of refractory affective disorders.

SURGERY

Copeland JG: Cardiac transplantation. ***Curr Probl Surg*** **25:613–672, September 1988.**

▶ This review emphasizes that the 2-year survival for patients with cardiac grafts ranges from 80% to 90% and is among the best for any organ graft. It is another example of the effect of cyclosporine therapy and addresses the important issues of improved cardiac preservation in the artificial heart and the possibility in the future of using xenographs.

Henderson JM, Warren WD: Portal hypertension. ***Curr Probl Surg*** **25:155–223, March 1988.**

▶ The contributions of Dr. Warren and the Emory group to our understanding of portal hypertension are unparalleled. It is laudatory that a surgeon who has had the procedure named for him has reported that the procedure should no longer represent the first line of therapy for acutely bleeding varices.

Nalesnik MA, Makowka L, Starzl TE: The diagnosis and treatment of posttransplant lymphoproliferative disorders. ***Curr Probl Surg*** **25:371–472, June 1988.**

▶ Dr. Chan, who is referred to extensively in the references, has focused on the development of these cell lymphomas and lymphoproliferative disorders in patients who are chronically immunosuppressed. The present review provides an updated and in-depth consideration of the problem and focuses appropriately on oncogene expression. The issue of spontaneous regression of these tumors, consequent to reduction of the immunosuppression, is particularly interesting.

Perry JF: Injuries of the spleen. ***Curr Probl Surg*** **25:757–859, December 1988.**

▶ Refinements in the diagnosis and treatment of splenic trauma have modified our attitudes significantly. Consideration of the relative applicability of computed tomography and radionuclide scanning and peritoneal lavage is crucial. An appreciation of the problem with overwhelming postsplenectomy infection, particularly in children, has led to a significant percentage of these forms of splenic trauma being treated nonoperatively. In adults, splenectomy is reported more frequently and is associated with a lower incidence of severe postsplenectomy infection. We continue to caution our surgeons that if there is any question as to whether the spleen should be removed to effect hemostasis, it should be removed, as the potential for continued hemorrhage is greater than that with postsplenectomy infection.

Rosenberg S: The development of new immunotherapies for the treatment of cancer using interleukin-2. ***Ann Surg*** **208:121–135, August 1988.**

▶ Immunotherapy represents the most modern adjuvant treatment of malignancy. The curtain on this episode of treatment has just risen. Modifications are expected to improve results.

Sunderland G, Carter DC: Clinical application of the cholecystokinin provocation test. ***Br J Surg*** **75:444–449, May 1988.**

▶ The assessment of patients with biliary tract pain but no demonstrable gallstones remains difficult. The efficacy of the cholecystokinin (CCK) provocative test to determine which patients will benefit from cholecystectomy is open to question, as the authors point out. Recently, Rhodes et al. (*Br J Surg* 75:951, 1988) carried out a prospective, placebo-controlled, crossover study of the patients who experienced pain after CCK. This work reported that only 9% did not benefit from cholecystectomy. These findings compare well with statistics of patients undergoing cholecystectomy for uncomplicated calculous gallbladder disease.

Warshaw AL, et al: Pancreatic cancer in 1988. ***Ann Surg*** **208:541–553, November 1988.**

▶ This excellent review addresses the major issues under consideration today. The survival figures for patients with carcinoma of the pancreas remain dismal; pancreatectomy has aided little, and very few surgons apply this procedure. There is really no uniform satisfaction with the use of adjuvant radiation therapy, and the article points out that the local survival time was unaltered. I agree with the authors that at a time when we have reduced the operative mortality to extremely low levels, a case can be made for an aggressive approach of resection in an appropriate subset of patients. That subset comprises younger patients who have no evidence of metastases or no resectable lesions.

JOURNAL SUBSCRIPTION APPENDIX

Of the more than 20,000 medical journals published weekly, bi-weekly, monthly, and quarterly, how do you choose which ones to read? They all have something to offer, but how do you decide which gives you the kind of information you need in the most efficient manner? It's mostly trial and error, although most of the trials have already been conducted by your peer group. Here is a list of what may be the core curriculum of medical journals, as well as information on how to subscribe to the journals.

Must Reads

American Journal of Diseases of Children
American Medical Association
535 North Dearborn Street
Chicago, IL 60610
Monthly
Students/Residents: $24.00

American Journal of Medicine
Cahners Publishing Company
44 Cook Street
Denver, CO 80206-5191
Monthly
Students/Interns/Residents: $31.50

American Journal of Obstetrics & Gynecology
The C. V. Mosby Company
11830 Westline Industrial Drive
St. Louis, MO 63141
Monthly
Students/Residents: $38.00

American Journal of Surgery
Cahners Publishing Company
44 Cook Street
Denver, CO 80206-5191
Monthly
Students/Residents: $34.50

Annals of Internal Medicine
4200 Pine Street
Philadelphia, PA 19104
Twice a month

Students: $30.50
Residents: $45.75

Annals of Surgery
J.B. Lippincott - Subscriber Services
Downsville Pike, Route 3
Box 20-B
Hagerstown, MD 21740
Monthly
Students/Residents: $39.00

Archives of General Psychiatry
American Medical Association
535 North Dearborn Street
Chicago, IL 60610
Monthly
Students/Residents: $25.00

Journal of the American Medical Association
Circulation and Fulfillment
535 North Dearborn Street
Chicago, IL 60610
Weekly
Students/Residents: $33.00 (1 year), $58.50 (2 years)

Journal of Pediatrics
The C. V. Mosby Company
11830 Westline Industrial Drive
St. Louis, MO 63146-3318
Monthly
Students/Residents: $30.00 (US), $53.00 (Can & Mex)

New England Journal of Medicine
Customer Service Department
P.O. Box 803
Waltham, MA 02254-0803
Weekly
Students: $37.00
Interns/Residents: $43.00

Obstetrics & Gynecology
Elsevier Science Publishing Company
52 Vanderbilt Avenue
New York, NY 10017

Monthly
Interns/Residents: $58.00

Pediatrics
American Academy of Pediatrics
P.O. Box 927
Elk Grove Village, IL 60009-0927
Monthly
Students/Free to Residents through Mead Johnson: $34.00

Surgery, Gynecology & Obstetrics
54 East Erie Street
Chicago, IL 60611
Monthly
Students/Residents: $30.00

Other Important Journals

Academic Medicine
Association of American Medical Colleges
Suite 200
One DuPont Circle, NW
Washington, DC 20036
Students: $30.00

American Journal of Cardiology
Cahners Publishing Company
44 Cook Street
Denver, CO 80206-5800
Monthly
Students/Interns/Residents: $33.00 (US), $85.00 (Canada)

Archives of Internal Medicine
American Medical Association
535 North Dearborn Street
Chicago, IL 60610
Monthly
Students/Residents: $21.00

British Medical Journal
British Medical Association
P.O. Box 295
London WC1H 9TE
England

Weekly
All: $164.00

Circulation
American Heart Association, Inc.
7320 Greenville Avenue
Dallas, TX 75231
Monthly
Students/Interns/Residents: $42.00 (US), $66.50 (Canada and Mexico)

Lancet
Williams & Wilkins Company
428 East Preston Street
Baltimore, MD 21202
Weekly
Students: $35.00
Interns/Residents: $48.50

Medicine
Williams & Wilkins Company
428 East Preston Street
Baltimore, MD 21202
Bimonthly
Students/Interns/Residents: $30.00

Science
American Association for the Advancement of Science
1333 H Street, NW
Washington, DC 20005
Weekly
Student rates on request

Author and Subject Index

A

C

Author and Subject Index

E

F

G

H

I

M

N

O

P

Q

R

T

U

V

W

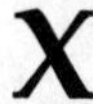

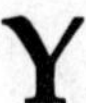

Z

THE 1990 YEAR BOOK® SERIES

As you define and refine your areas of interest, we thought you would like to know about other titles in the YEAR BOOK series. To learn more about the series or a particular YEAR BOOK title, you can call us toll-free at 1-800-622-5410 or write us at 200 North LaSalle Street, Suite 2500, Chicago, Illinois 60601.

Year Book Medical Publishers (est. 1901) was the first company to offer abstracts of articles enhanced by expert editorial commentary in an annual book format. YEAR BOOKS are now published in nearly 40 specialties.

Year Book of Anesthesia®
Drs. Miller, Kirby, Ostheimer, Roizen, and Stoelting

Year Book of Cardiology®
Drs. Schlant, Collins, Engle, Frye, Kaplan, and O'Rourke

Year Book of Critical Care Medicine®
Drs. Rogers and Parrillo

Year Book of Dentistry®
Drs. Meskin, Ackerman, Kennedy, Leinfelder, Matukas, and Rovin

Year Book of Dermatology®
Drs. Sober and Fitzpatrick

Year Book of Diagnostic Radiology®
Drs. Bragg, Hendee, Keats, Kirkpatrick, Miller, Osborn, and Thompson

Year Book of Digestive Diseases®
Drs. Greenberger and Moody

Year Book of Drug Therapy®
Drs. Hollister and Lasagna

Year Book of Emergency Medicine®
Dr. Wagner

Year Book of Endocrinology®
Drs. Bagdade, Braverman, Halter, Horton, Kannan, Korenman, Molitch, Morley, Odell, Rogol, Ryan, and Sherwin

Year Book of Family Practice®
Drs. Rakel, Avant, Driscoll, Prichard, and Smith

Year Book of Geriatrics and Gerontology®
Drs. Beck, Abrass, Burton, Cummings, Makinodan, and Small

Year Book of Hand Surgery®
Drs. Dobyns, Chase, and Amadio

Year Book of Hematology®
Drs. Spivak, Bell, Ness, Quesenberry, and Wiernik

Year Book of Infectious Diseases®
Drs. Wolff, Barza, Keusch, Klempner, and Snydman

Year Book of Infertility
Drs. Mishell, Paulsen, and Lobo

Year Book of Medicine®
Drs. Rogers, Des Prez, Cline, Braunwald, Greenberger, Wilson, Epstein, and Malawista

Year Book of Neonatal and Perinatal Medicine
Drs. Klaus and Fanaroff

Year Book of Neurology and Neurosurgery®
Drs. Currier and Crowell

Year Book of Nuclear Medicine®
Drs. Hoffer, Gore, Gottschalk, Sostman, Zaret, and Zubal

Year Book of Obstetrics and Gynecology®
Drs. Mishell, Kirschbaum, and Morrow

Year Book of Occupational and Environmental Medicine
Drs. Emmett, Brooks, Harris, and Schenker

Year Book of Oncology
Drs. Young, Longo, Ozols, Simone, Steele, and Weichselbaum

Year Book of Ophthalmology®
Drs. Laibson, Adams, Augsburger, Benson, Cohen, Eagle, Flanagan, Nelson, Reinecke, Sergott and Wilson

Year Book of Orthopedics®
Drs. Sledge, Poss, Cofield, Frymoyer, Griffin, Hansen, Johnson, Springfield, and Weiland

Year Book of Otolaryngology—Head and Neck Surgery®
Drs. Bailey and Paparella

Year Book of Pathology and Clinical Pathology®
Drs. Brinkhous, Dalldorf, Grisham, Langdell, and McLendon

Year Book of Pediatrics®
Drs. Oski and Stockman

Year Book of Plastic, Reconstructive, and Aesthetic Surgery
Drs. Miller, Bennett, Haynes, Hoehn, McKinney, and Whitaker

Year Book of Podiatric Medicine and Surgery®
Dr. Jay

Year Book of Psychiatry and Applied Mental Health®
Drs. Talbott, Frances, Frances, Freedman, Meltzer, Schowalter, and Yudofsky

Year Book of Pulmonary Disease®
Drs. Green, Loughlin, Michael, Mulshine, Peters, Terry, Tockman, and Wise

Year Book of Speech, Language, and Hearing
Drs. Bernthal, Hall, and Tomblin

Year Book of Sports Medicine®
Drs. Shephard, Eichner, Sutton, and Torg, Col. Anderson, and Mr. George

Year Book of Surgery®
Drs. Schwartz, Jonasson, Peacock, Shires, Spencer, and Thompson

Year Book of Urology®
Drs. Gillenwater and Howards

Year Book of Vascular Surgery®
Drs. Bergan and Yao

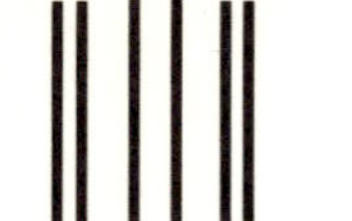

NO POSTAGE
NECESSARY
IF MAILED
IN THE
UNITED STATES

BUSINESS REPLY MAIL

FIRST CLASS PERMIT No. 762 CHICAGO, ILLINOIS

POSTAGE WILL BE PAID BY ADDRESSEE

Year Book Medical Publishers
200 North LaSalle Street
Chicago, IL 60601-9981